FOREWORD BY DR. DONALD M. JOY

Talking with Your Kids About

the Birds *and the* Bees

A Guide for Parents and Counselors
to Help Kids from 4 to 18
Develop Healthy Sexual Attitudes

SCOTT TALLEY

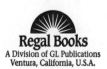

Regal Books
A Division of GL Publications
Ventura, California, U.S.A.

Published by Regal Books
A Division of GL Publications
Ventura, California 93006
Printed in U.S.A.

Library of Congress Cataloging-in-Publication Data

Scott, Talley.
    Talking with your kids about the birds and the bees: a guide for parents and counselors to help kids from 4 to 18 develop healthy sexual attitudes / Scott Talley.
        p. cm.
    Includes bibliographical references.
    ISBN 0-8307-1398-0
    1. Sex instruction. 2. Parenting. 3. Sex—Religious aspects—Christianity. I. Title.
HQ57.S36 1990
649'.65—dc20   90-8589
                                                                     CIP

Rights for publishing this book in other languages are contracted by Gospel Literature International (GLINT) foundation. GLINT also provides technical help for the adaptation, translation, and publishing of Bible study resources and books in scores of languages worldwide. For further information, contact GLINT, Post Office Box 488, Rosemead, California, 91770, U.S.A., or the publisher.

CONTENTS

ACKNOWLEDGMENTS

This book is the result of much work by many people. I am indebted to those who made this task bearable for me.

To the Christians at the Crestview Church of Christ—thanks for encouraging me for 14 years.

To my mentors, Lynn Anderson and Glenn Austin—Lynn made God's word come alive in all its richness and grace. Glenn taught me about stretching myself and the need to be a suffering servant.

To my secretary, Helen McDowell, who typed and worked on the manuscript—she labored well above the call of duty.

To my editor and friend, Ron Durham—Ron believed in me from the start. His help and encouragement strengthened me and helped me believe in myself.

And lastly and most importantly, this book is dedicated to my wife, Linda. Her many hours spent in editing and correcting the manuscript made this work possible. She provided me with spiritual wisdom and constant encouragement, and her name deserves to be on the cover with mine.

FOREWORD

Has Scott Talley got good news for you!

In fact, his book is good news for everyone, for we are all running scared these days. In the good old days we could pray a lot or cross our fingers and count on our kids' naivete to keep them virginal and clean until they were full grown. And even when that silent strategy failed—which it often did—we could wring our hands, point accusing fingers at failed kids and feel sorry for their "victim" parents.

But today we know we are all victims. The seducers are everywhere—and they want our kids. They distort data, making the kids feel media pressure to be cool by joining that "sexually active majority"—a majority which is partly fiction but entirely a creation of the hype crowd.

For some of the charlatans, money is to be made in seducing our kids through the sex magazines, movies and videos they target to the young. At the same time, we all experience a rippling sort of public sexual arousal through the tabloids that titillate us with headlines and news stories of the sexual misadventures of famous personalities along with accounts of everything else sexual that is falling out of the closet.

And many parents—remembering how naive they were in their teens at the time of their own emerging sexuality and its accompanying energy—now get midlife sexual kicks out of coaching, cheering on or giving nodding permission for their kids to become active. But this apparent, free-ride sexual adventure only works with folks who have a short memory. Sexually active teens soon turn out to be afraid of or incapable of making marriage commitments. And those that do try prove to be high-risk partners for those seeking exclusively bonded, lifelong intimacy in marriage.

Those fearful but monogamous lovers who become "living togethers" are twice as likely to divorce when they marry. Paul Pearsall nailed it honestly in his recent best-seller, *Super Marital Sex: Loving for Life*, when he cautioned that sex is not like tennis. Practice does not make perfect; it only leads to more practice. And the bottom line, he insists, is that we simply must tell our young people to abstain from sexual intercourse before marriage.

All the bad news about what is out there sexually in our culture is, of course, increasingly complicated by the numerically exploding incidences of sexually transmitted diseases among unsuspecting playful folk, but particularly so by that silent, fatal sleeper, AIDS.

That's why this new book by Scott Talley is good news. He has written a bright good word to make us wise and competent as parents in this drama that has a sexually explicit script being written for us and our kids by other folks and forces. These lines by Talley recapture human sexuality for God and grace and good.

Most parents past 30 today feel dumb when faced with explicit sexual issues. We didn't feel dumb, of course, at 15, but a ripening maturity has shown us our ignorance. We didn't understand our own sexuality, so how could we possibly pretend to understand sexuality in our kids?

This book will free us from those dumb feelings and help build our parental self-respect. Thanks to Talley, we can know the truth about human sexuality, and the truth will make us more comfortable because he puts the vocabulary of honesty and sex-positive hope right there before us.

To encourage you at an even deeper level, know that you

don't need to be running scared. Today's families have the wonderful option of pulling together into a sort of emotional and spiritual huddle. Putting their heads together in a friendship pact, they can peer over their shoulders and scout the opposition as it flexes its muscle. These families can know that family honesty, commitment and time together is the combination that wins in today's war against sexual exploitation and deception.

The best family research of the last 30 years confirms exactly what Christian parents have always believed was true—that three simple, intentional family practices can anchor a family:
- a commitment to each other,
- a love of cohesive times together, and
- a resolve never to be a "missing person," always leaving word about to be found in an emergency.

These simple "huddle" strategies ensure a 97.1 percent rate in risk-proofing kids against their being devastated in a world gone crazy. And remember this simple agenda for breakfast and daily launching: huddle up and give each other to God's protection for the day.

We have every reason to believe that if we add prayer to honesty, grounding our faithfulness to God in our commitment to each other, and remain accountable to each other in unconditional Christian love, we might even cut into that 2.9 percent margin of failure and loss.

So take courage and be glad that we live in a moral universe where choices matter. Get smart with the Talley script in your mind and on your lips. And stay relaxed and affirming as you huddle your family every day to celebrate God's surrounding grace which empowers us all to live every day as agents of light in the world.

—Donald M. Joy, Ph.D.
Professor of Human Development
Ray and Mary Jo West Chair of Christian Education
Asbury Theological Seminary
Wilmore, Kentucky

INTRODUCTION

During seventeen years in youth ministry I have observed many changes in our society and culture. Values, beliefs, ideals and morals are all being redefined as a secular society gropes for its moorings. Churches and families have also felt the impact of our rapidly changing moral environment. It is becoming increasingly difficult for families to develop moral sense in our swiftly changing world.

Nowhere is this more visible than in our society's preoccupation with sex. Madison Avenue advertisers use sex to sell everything from automobiles to children's clothes. It is almost impossible to escape daily exposure to sexual references in the media. This cultural preoccupation not only affects society as a whole, but especially harms children and adolescents. Young people between the ages of thirteen and nineteen do not have sufficient emotional, physical and spiritual maturity to deal with the complex issues of human sexuality they are faced with. Our society's new sexual morality presents Christian parents with many challenges as they attempt to rear in the words of Tipper Gore, "P. G. kids in an X-rated society."

It's a Different Ball Game

The fact that our society seems to be encouraging sexual immorality more and more is having rather dramatic effects.

Consider these statistics published in a recent book on teenage sexuality:

- Research shows that the average age for first having sex is 15 for girls and 14 for boys.
- The New York polling firm Audit and Survey Research study showed that 57 percent of high school students and 79 percent of college students had lost their virginity.
- Among thirteen-year-old boys, 20 percent have touched a girl's breast, 54 percent of fourteen-year-old boys have engaged in breast play.
- This year more than 1.1 million teenage girls will become pregnant.[1]

One would hope that the behavior of Christian teens would follow a significantly different trend. But this is not the case. A recent study of teenagers in evangelical churches revealed:

- By eighteen years of age, 43 percent have had sexual intercourse.
- Fondling breasts is considered to be morally acceptable at times by 32 percent.
- And 32 percent also see fondling genitals as sometimes morally acceptable.
- About 35 percent could not state that premarital sexual intercourse is always morally unacceptable.[2]
- Between 45 and 50 percent of evangelical Christian youth are involved in sexual activity. Studies generally show that the percentage of sexually active Christian youth is about ten points behind the percentage of all teens.

It should be noted, of course, that the accuracy of all statistics is dependent on the size of the sample and the method of sampling, the instrument used to obtain the information and many other factors. For example, statistics indicating that 50 percent of all teens between the ages of fifteen and nineteen are sexually active, are somewhat misleading. Parents of younger teens should know that not until age nineteen for women and eighteen for men do the actual figures reach 50 percent. There is good news, too, for kids who value church involvement. For instance, adolescents who consider youth ministry extremely helpful have an 80 percent virginity rate compared to a 58 percent rate among adolescents who consider youth ministry unhelpful.[3]

The majority of the statistics I have cited, of course, indicate that sexual activity among teens has been steadily rising for several years.

Why do such figures surprise us? For one thing, most parents of today's teenagers were reared in the 1960s and 1970s. It is still very difficult for many of us to understand fully just how much sexual attitudes have changed since our own teen years. One reason may be that we do not have contact with significant numbers of adolescents and we have limited access to their world. Another contributing factor is the strong reluctance we parents have to believe that our children are involved in sexual misconduct. Sexual activity among our children is too emotionally painful for many Christian parents to contemplate; therefore, we simply ignore it. But this means ignoring many teens! Parents desperately need to understand that for teenagers, sexual pressure and temptation have increased drastically.

When I first began working as a youth minister in the early '70s, comparatively little of my time was spent counseling teens regarding sexual misconduct. By the late '70s and early '80s, however, things were changing and far more of my time was being consumed by this. I answered the phone late one evening to hear the voice of one of the teenage girls in my youth group. She told me she had just returned from the clinic and was pregnant. She asked if I would accompany her to tell her parents. I was shocked, not only because this was my first experience of this kind, but also because this was "one of our own." This young lady came from a dedicated Christian family; both her mother and father were Sunday School teachers. This was a good girl. But she was pregnant! It is apparent that sexual misconduct, sometimes resulting in pregnancy, is occurring with alarming regularity among young people from all types of families.

A more recent example will help illustrate the rapid sexual changes occurring in our society. A few months ago I found my fourteen-year-old son burning a picture of his most recent girlfriend. Most fourteen-year-olds change boyfriends and girlfriends about as often as they change clothes, so I was not overly concerned about the change itself. But my son is not usually given to such severe emotional reactions, so I went into his room and asked why he was so upset with this young lady.

He said, "I'm sorry I burned her picture, but I was very upset with her and it seemed like a good idea."

Then I asked him to tell me why he was so upset.

"Well, Dad," he said, "I found out that she went to an unchaperoned party this past weekend and had sex with a guy."

I cautioned him about unsubstantiated rumors and the need to protect the reputation of the young lady, but he interrupted me.

"Dad," he replied, "she admitted it!"

That experience allowed my son and me to have some very meaningful conversations about sex, temptation, parties, and many other subjects. But I was sad for him and for this fourteen-year-old girl who perhaps unknowingly has created a multitude of problems at such a tender age.

Dear John

In the fall of 1988 a new situation comedy appeared on NBC. "Dear John" focuses on the life of a man whose wife has unexpectedly left him. A large part of the show portrays a divorce recovery support group. The members of this group exchange personal stories and furnish support for one another. During one episode, the star related a problem he anticipated having to face. He told the group members about how he had lost his virginity at the age of fifteen, to a woman several years older. He recalled, with much fondness, very specific details of that night long ago.

When the group inquired about the potential problem, he

told them that the woman had called and requested a meeting. His assumption was that this older woman wanted to renew the sexual relationship. He was not very excited about the possibility because she was now a grandmother. A substantial part of the episode dealt with his attempts to evade what he thought was to be a sexual encounter with an older woman.

The support group leader endeavored to shame the star. She explained that since this woman had helped him at a tender, unlovable age, he should be willing to help her at a time in her life when she needed help and support. Not once during the entire half-hour program was the morality of either of these extramarital encounters discussed. Sex between these two individuals was apparently viewed as nothing more than providing a helping hand to an emotionally needy person. It was portrayed as neither moral nor immoral.

The way in which sexual morality is being eroded by the media, especially television, is alarming. For example, in the '50s when Lucille Ball on "I Love Lucy" was expecting a child, the word "pregnant" was not allowed on the air. In the '60s Rob and Laura on "The Dick Van Dyke Show," slept in twin beds. In less than two decades television has shifted from depicting married couples in twin beds to openly encouraging extramarital sex for the purpose of, among other things, repaying old debts and improving self-esteem in the middle-aged. Times have certainly changed! Recent research reported by author Josh McDowell estimates that in one year the average person views approximately 9,230 sex acts or implied sex acts on television. Of that sexual activity, 81 percent is outside the commitment of marriage. McDowell also reports that television portrays six times more extramarital sex than sex between spouses.[4]

What Are We Telling Our Kids?

Most information and counseling given to adolescents regarding sexual activity emphasizes disease and pregnancy prevention. These are admirable goals, but almost no teaching regarding the *morality* of premarital sex is given. In his recent book *Parents, Kids and Sexual Integrity*, Donald M. Joy says:

> The current preoccupation with pregnancy preventative and disease control tends to miss the heart of the sexual issue. Safe sex in the face of today's AIDS epidemic trivializes sexual activity and guarantees that today's practices will remain forever outside and apart from the meaning of sexual intimacy and communication. Abortion and pregnancy control suggests that as long as there is no pregnancy...or at least no baby...anything is appropriate to the amoral game of frustrated adolescents who only want to play house on weeknights and weekends. They are the victims in this drama of premature sexual intimacy in our confused culture. My plea here is both to today's parents and to today's youth who will form tomorrow's households to live out a vision very different from that of a promiscuous culture.[5]

I echo Dr. Joy's plea. Certainly children and adolescents must be warned about the damaging physical consequences of sexual activity, but children must also be taught that premarital sex violates and defiles the sanctity of God's laws. In other words, they should learn that premarital sex is morally wrong. Do not be afraid to view the teaching of sexual morality as an end in itself.

Most Christian parents feel the need to teach their children to abstain from sexual activity. But they also need to teach them a healthy, wholesome, godly attitude toward their sexuality. We must provide our children with accurate, adequate sexual information and motivation rooted in a consistent and biblical framework. The premise of this book is that, even in today's sexually immoral culture, parents can effectively model and teach sexual morality.

Jump in with Both Feet!

Many aspects of sexuality will be discussed in this book. My objective is to equip parents with knowledge and information which children need in learning about human sexuality. In addition, you will learn *how* and *when* to use the information. The topics covered include:

• Understanding and accepting your own sexuality
• Sources of our children's sexual information
• How to communicate effectively with our children
• How to become an askable parent
• Family structure and discipline
• When, where and how to talk to our children about sex
• Specific factual information appropriate for each age
• Specifically age-related topics: puberty, menstruation, masturbation, birth control, dating, socially transmitted diseases
• At each age category the effects of self-esteem, peer pressure, and stress on sexuality will be examined.

It should also be noted that while subjects such as communication and discipline may not directly relate to sexuality, they promote a healthy family atmosphere without which instruction on sexual matters would be very difficult. This book is the result of research and study of competent authorities, both secular and Christian, in the field of sex education, and of almost twenty years of ministry with parents and young people making decisions in a Christian framework about their own sexuality.

Remember as you engage in this important and sometimes frightening task, that you occupy a unique position in the life of your child. Your relationship, based on your love and knowledge as a parent, enables you to communicate and teach your children a biblical view of sex better than anyone else. And if they are to acquire a godly, moral understanding and appreciation for human sexuality...you must teach your children!

Chapter 1

WE'RE GONNA TALK WITH OUR KIDS ABOUT WHAT?

The mere thought of talking to their children about sex renders many parents totally speechless. Even the most confident, self-assured parents may shudder when contemplating a "facts-of-life" talk with their twelve-year-old son or daughter. But regardless of fear and sweaty palms, this is a task you cannot get out of. Grace Ketterman states in her book, *How to Teach Your Child About Sex*, "every parent teaches his or her child about sex, sometimes without even realizing it. Like it or not, it's a fact of life. A parent may do it in a well planned fashion or haphazardly. Nevertheless, each child learns sexual lessons from his parents."[1]

The Institute for Family Research and Education takes the same position: "Parents are the sex educators of their children whether they do it well or badly. Silence teaches no less eloquently than words."[2]

Parental Sexuality

But before leaping headlong into educating your children about sex, you should take time for some self-evaluation. Such evaluation is necessary because attitudes, values and beliefs concerning our own sexuality dramatically affect what we teach our children about sex. Perhaps a good starting place would be to simply ask yourself "Am I comfortable with my own sexuality?" Parents are often embarrassed or uncomfortable talking to their children about sex because they are not comfortable with their own sexuality. Surgeon General C. Everett Koop believes that the best thing parents can do for their children is to feel comfortable about their own sexuality.[3] Unhappy sexual attitudes can affect not only what you teach, but also what you model. Remember parents' behavior and attitudes toward sex and marriage teach children more than words do. Children learn a great deal about sex and sexual matters by simply watching and observing their parents, so parents are teaching values and beliefs both verbally and nonverbally.

First of all, parents need to accept themselves and their mates physically. In other words, be comfortable with your body and appearance and the body and appearance of your mate. This will communicate physical acceptance to your children and make it easier for them to accept themselves physically.

Parents should communicate to their children that they love each other not just platonically, but sexually. Children should be taught that God created us as sexual beings, and that within the context of marriage sexual expressions are normal and healthy. Such communication is important because young people often grow up without an awareness that their parents are sexually attracted to each other. A survey among college students revealed that many of them could not imagine their parents having sex. Parents should let their children know in appropriate ways that they love each other and enjoy their sexual relationship. If children see their parents treat sex in a wholesome, normal way as God intended, they will be more apt to emulate their parents and do the same.[4]

Learning to handle emotions openly and positively can be helpful as parents attempt to model healthy, sexual attitudes. This is true because the interaction of our sexual attitudes and emotions is very important. Many people do not enjoy a good sex life because they have been conditioned to deny their emotions in every aspect of their lives. And when emotions are left unexpressed or misunderstood, they begin to create a barrier between partners. Many adults have developed a habit of protecting vulnerable feelings such as hurts, disappointments and loneliness with a facade of anger. Such a habit on the part of one or both spouses can interfere with positive sexual feelings and attitudes. Learning to communicate one's feelings openly and honestly not only contributes to solving marital problems, but also models positive, helpful attitudes to children. Of course, a complex subject like emotional openness should not be trivialized and learning it can be a long, difficult process. My point, however, is that your emotions can and do affect your sexuality as well as what you model to your children.

Our attitudes, values, and beliefs concerning sexuality are influenced by our past experiences. Childhood experiences and parental influence affect individuals well into their adult lives. We are all influenced by our past.

Sorting out values and feelings is an interesting process. It is also a sensitive and fragile task, requiring honesty with yourself. Although this self-examination can be painful, getting in touch with your feelings and clarifying your values is both necessary and rewarding.

It may be helpful to think of the process as a "journey of exploration" into your inner self. Ideally, at the end of this imaginary journey you will have a clearer picture of your own feelings, values, and attitudes concerning sex. The journey may trigger deeply buried emotions and recollections of painful experiences, but by remembering and reliving these events of the past you will be better enabled to empathize with your children. In addition, from a practical standpoint, you may remember negative examples from your own childhood sex education experiences that can be avoided with your children.

It may be easier for you to take this journey if you can get someone to read the questions for you while you sit with your eyes closed. Whether you are reading the questions yourself or having them read to you, proceed slowly, taking time to collect all your thoughts after each question. It will be helpful to find a place where you are comfortable and where you will not be disturbed. Please remember that the purpose of this journey and these questions is to help you not only to focus on your own values, feelings and attitudes, but also to define your goals and objectives in teaching your children about sex.

The Journey

Close your eyes and think back to your childhood. Think back as far as you can.

- What was the first question about sex you can remember asking your parents? How did they respond?
- From what sources (parents, friends, books) did you first learn the basic facts about reproduction and intercourse?
- How did you feel upon acquiring this information?
- Were you ever punished or made to feel guilty or ashamed because of childhood curiosity about your own or a playmate's body ("playing doctor," or "physical exam")?
- Were you informed by your parents about menstruation, nocturnal emissions and masturbation?
- How open and honest were your parents in discussing sex with you? Did either, or both, of your parents act embarrassed or angry when discussing sexual matters?
- As you entered your late teens did you have all the sexual information you felt you needed or desired?
- Did you feel guilty as a result of your sexual feelings?
- Was most of your sexual information about physical and/or biological aspects? Were you ever given information about the emotional, psychological and spiritual aspects of sex?

- How was love and affection shown or demonstrated by your parents (either to you or to each other).

Open your eyes. What have you learned about yourself and your sexual attitudes?

As you continue in this evaluation process, it is important for you and your spouse to communicate with each other about sexual needs and problems. Such frank communication is important because if a husband and wife do not feel free to talk to each other about their sexuality, they will not feel free to talk about the subject with their children. To gain this comfort requires open, honest communication, not only between spouses, but also between parents and children. In your role as a modeling, teaching parent, open and intimate communication with your children is especially important. This personal touch in the area of parent-child communication is very effective because what your children learn is as much caught as taught.

> If communication has been open with children and if the parents themselves believe that sex should be connected with love, then teens are less likely to be effected by what peers are doing.[5]

In other words, your influence can be dramatically increased by close, intimate communication.

Sometimes one or both partners in a marriage may be troubled by persistent, ongoing sexual problems. If this is your situation, seek professional help. Parents cannot offer their children appropriate sex education if all their energy and attention is consumed with their own sexual problems.

The focus of this book is not marital sexual problems, and the preceding paragraphs are not intended to be exhaustive or all-inclusive suggestions. The focal point is that parents model sexual attitudes and values to their children daily and that parental goals of effective sex education can best be accomplished by healthy, wholesome, positive attitudes regarding sexuality in general and your own sexuality specifically.

Earlier I gave you some questions to help you clarify early

influences on your own sexual attitudes. Try the same procedure with the questions that follow. They will help you identify your feelings about your role in your children's sexual education.

Close your eyes now and think about these questions:
- Do you have difficulty talking to your children about sex?
- Do you feel that you have adequate information to discuss sexual matters with your children? In other words, do you know how and when to talk to your children about sex?
- Are you comfortable with your own sexuality?
- Do you feel you are an approachable and askable parent?
- Do you think your children really want to discuss sex with you?
- What are the sources of your children's sexual information?
- What kind of perspective about sexuality and relationships do you think your children are developing by watching your example?
- What are your major concerns and fears as you think about teaching your children about sex?

Open your eyes. How are you feeling after pondering these questions? A little nervous? During the next few chapters your courage and confidence will hopefully increase as you acquire information that will improve your ability to talk to your children about sex.

Not All Bad News

Earlier I mentioned several very disturbing facts regarding teenage sex and pregnancy. And these statistics represent only the tip of the iceberg. Page after page of distressing and troublesome data concerning sexual immorality among adolescents could be catalogued. However, not all the news is bad. A great deal of recent research is discovering that family closeness, openness and religious training can have very beneficial effects not only on sexual practices of adolescents, but also on other deviant behavior. For example, Merton and Irene Strommen, noted researchers and authors, state in their book *Five Cries of Parents*:

> Adolescents in a close family unit are the ones most likely to say no to drug use, premarital sexual activity, and other anti-social and alienating behavior. They are also the ones most likely to adopt high moral standards, develop the ability to make and keep friends, embrace a religious faith, and involve themselves in helping activities. All of these characteristics pertaining to adolescents from close families are significant—which means that the evidence cannot be attributed to mere chance.[6]

In addition:

> A study of teenage sex-related values and behavior was done by sociologist Brent Miller at Utah State University and reported in "The Family's Role in Adolescent Sexual Behavior." Miller discovered that the more openly parents discussed their sex-related values and beliefs with teens, the less their children displayed either negative sexual attitudes or promiscuous sexual behavior. He also shows that teens who learned sexual facts from parents were significantly less likely to be sexually active than those who first heard about sex from their friends.[7]

These researchers are telling parents that family closeness, as expressed, among other ways, through open, honest sex education, can promote abstinence from sexual activity. This is good news!

Myths About Sex Education

Distinguishing between fact and fiction in the area of sex education can at times be extremely difficult. To a large extent this difficulty is compounded by the controversial nature of the subject. It is, however, very important for parents to be able to differentiate between facts and myths in the areas of sex education. With this in mind, pause in your reading and take this quick true/false test. After answering the questions, read on and discover which are facts and which are myths!

1. In today's enlightened culture, adolescents   T   F
already possess adequate sexual information.
2. Teenagers know more about sex than   T   F
most of their parents.
3. Sexual knowledge is harmful to children   T   F
and adolescents.
4. Children do not want to talk to their   T   F
parents about sex.
5. In order to talk effectively to children   T   F
about sex, parents need specific, scientific
technical information.
6. Parents must be completely comfortable   T   F
about all aspects of sexuality in order
to be effective with their children.
7. It is possible to give a child too much   T   F
information.
8. Parental mistakes in sex education   T   F
are irreversibly damaging to the child.

Hopefully, you answered false to all the above questions, since they represent some popularly held myths about sex education. Take, for example, the first two questions. Research shockingly reveals that adolescents are actually ignorant about critical sexual issues. In an important 1976 Johns Hopkins study of adolescent girls, only 41 percent knew when in the menstrual cycle the risk of conception was greatest.[8] Granted, from their exposure to adult fare on television and in the printed media, today's children know many more sex-related words than their parents and grandparents did at the same age, but David Elkind, in his insightful book *The Hurried Child* labels this phenomenon "pseudo-sophistication."

Children today know more than they understand.
They are able to talk about nuclear fission, tube

worms at 20,000 fathoms, and the space shuttle; and they seem knowledgeable about sex and crime. But much of the knowledge is largely verbal. Adults, however, are often taken in by this pseudo-sophistication and treat children as if they were as knowledgeable as they sound. Ironically, the pseudo-sophistication, which is the effect of television hurrying children, encourage parents and adults to hurry them even more. But children who sound, behave, and look like adults still feel and think like children.[9]

Today's youth simply do not know enough about sex. Furthermore, the facts they do possess are not clearly understood in the complex context of human sexuality. Children need

---

Evidence indicates that it is actually ignorance, not knowledge, that leads to promiscuous behavior.

---

help from their parents in order to give meaning and understanding to sexual words and sexual feelings.

Question 3 deals with whether or not sexual information is harmful to children and adolescents. Again, generally speaking, the answer is false. Information alone is not harmful. Those who subscribe to this myth hold the view that sexual knowledge in and of itself will promote inappropriate sexual behavior or promiscuity. They believe that if adolescents understand and know about sexual matters, they will engage in sexual activity. After several years of searching, I have yet to find reputable evidence (books, journals, articles or personal interviews) documenting the notion that children have been motivated toward promiscuous behavior by facts alone. The evidence indicates that it is actually ignorance, not knowledge, that leads to promiscuous behavior.

Question 4 relates to children's desire to talk to their parents about sex. The belief that children do not want to talk to their parents about sex is another myth. Although this may be true to some extent as children reach adolescence, even then this reluctance usually occurs only briefly and is related to typical adolescent behavior. Most children, especially pre-adolescents and older adolescents, welcome honest, frank discussions with their parents about sexual matters. We shall talk more about this later.

Question 5 applies to the parental myth of scientific or technical inadequacy. Some parents believe that they must be in command of specific, detailed sexual information in order to be helpful and effective communicators with their children. In fact most parents have adequate knowledge to teach their children about sexual matters. It is not necessary to be an M.D., Ph.D, or clinical psychologist in order to communicate sexual information to your children. Teaching children about sex in a moral and biblical context is vitally important and should be the legacy all Christian parents give to their children. As parents you need not be discouraged by this myth, for the technical information you need can be easily and quickly learned.

Question 6 concerns the myth that parents must be thoroughly comfortable with all phases of sexuality in order to be effective teachers to their children. Because of the complexity of human sexuality, few parents feel totally comfortable addressing the subject. But children will understand if parents admit uneasy feelings to their children and plunge ahead.

Questions 7 and 8 again apply to the subject of sexual knowledge and information. As we previously stated, knowledge alone is usually not harmful to children. Therefore, if parents make a mistake, it should be on the side of too much information, too soon—rather than too little, too late. Too much information does not over-stimulate children; it simply bores them.[10]

Parents should be encouraged by the resilience and forgiving nature of children. Because children are so flexible and forgiving, mistakes you may make in sex education are not fatal. The only response that may be disastrous or ruinous is not to respond at all.

It is extremely important that parents not be misled by sex education myths, and then fail to provide adequate sexual information to their children. If our children are to have quality sex education given in a moral and spiritual context, it must be provided in the home. So, parents, sweep aside the fantasies and fears and plunge ahead.

Sex education must begin at a very young age and continue as your children grow. In reality, the sex education of children

---

Sex education of children is an eighteen year course of love, insight and example. The goal is to provide children with accurate information and wholesome sexual attitudes based on God's principles and teachings.

---

is an eighteen year course of love, insight and example. Our goal is to provide children with accurate information and wholesome sexual attitudes based on God's principles and teachings. If you achieve this objective, you will be promoting healthy sexual attitudes and preparing your children for long-term godly marriages.

For Further Thought

1. Am I comfortable with my own sexuality? If not, why?
2. Do I accept my appearance, looks, and body, and do I accept my mate's appearance? Do I communicate acceptance?
3. Do I in an appropriate way convey to my children that I love and enjoy my mate sexually as well as platonically.
4. Do I openly and positively deal with and communicate emotions such as fear and anger? How do these emotions affect my sexuality?
5. What past experiences have influenced my sexual attitudes, values and beliefs?
6. Do I communicate my sexual needs and problems to my mate?

Chapter 2

WHERE DO THEY HEAR ALL THIS STUFF?

A friend of mine was driving home one night with his seven-year-old son. As they drove the boy asked if he could listen to the radio. The father turned on the radio and soon lost himself in his own thoughts. He was jerked back into reality by a remark from his son. The radio station was playing a popular teenage song of the day and the song contained the phrase "wild thing." The young boy proudly announced to his dad that he knew what "wild thing" really meant. His dad said, "Okay, son, tell me, what does it mean?" Becoming very quiet and mysterious, the seven-year-old confidently said, "'Wild thing', means sex!" The father was a bit stunned and paused a moment to collect his thoughts, but it was too late. His son had a follow-up question. "Dad," he said very seriously, "what is sex anyway?" My friend managed to compose himself and used this opportunity to teach an appropriate lesson on sex. As he was relating this humorous incident he asked me, "Where do they hear all this stuff?"

My friend's amusing tale caused me to pause and ask myself some very serious questions.

First, what are the sources of our children's sexual information? Where do they get the information, and from whom? And then, how accurate is this information?

Remember our goal is to provide children with wholesome sex education based on God's principles and teachings. Most of us agree that sex education remains primarily the responsibility of the parents. If we as parents are to discharge our responsibility as the primary sex educators of our children, we must know the sources and accuracy of our children's sexual information. Knowing the sources will help us determine who or what is influencing our children. When parents know the specific source of information and misinformation then counteraction is easier. Balancing or canceling negative influences will prove much easier if the influences are identifiable. It is also very important for parents to know the accuracy of their children's sexual information. Because much of what children learn about sex is false and inaccurate, a substantial amount of parental sex education may involve correcting erroneous facts and data.

Who Is Teaching Our Kids?

A recent poll of teenagers revealed some rather startling statistics concerning sexual information:

- Only 32 percent of girls and 15 percent of boys were informed about sex by their parents.
- 54 percent of boys and 42 percent of girls learned about sex from friends their own age.
- 15 percent pieced together information they had learned from other sources.
- 56 percent of these young people acquired their sex knowledge between the sixth and ninth grades and 18 percent learned about sex before the fifth grade.
- 88 percent of these young people felt they needed more

information about sex than they had received from their parents.[1]

These general statistics are not very encouraging. They do, however, emphasize that it is crucial for parents to have additional knowledge concerning who is teaching our kids.

In 1981 Hershal D. Thornburg of the Department of Educational Psychology at the University of Arizona, authored a study for the *Journal of Early Adolescence* titled "The Amount of Sex Information Learning Obtained During Early Adolescence." The purpose of this study was to investigate the sources, age and accuracy of sex information when it was initially obtained by adolescents.

Thornburg's article contains some facts that may be very interesting and beneficial to parents.

• Peers are the single most often cited source of sex information (37.1 percent).

• There are two categories where peers contribute more than 50 percent of the total information—petting and homosexuality. Sexual intercourse is another highly ranked area. In the areas regarding actual sexual behavior, peers seem to contribute the most information.

• The second most cited source of sex information is literature, including the media (21.9 percent). Abortion and seminal emissions are the two concepts learned primarily from the media.

• Fathers rank very low as a source of sexual information (2.2 percent). In fact, they rank below information gained from school and experience.

• Mothers rank third as a source of sex information (17.4 percent).

Thornburg's research also showed that in some areas males and females are likely to seek out different sources to learn sexual concepts. Females, for example, are more dependent on their mothers for information. According to the study, they obtain three times more information from their mothers than do their male counterparts. Males, on the other hand, are clearly more dependent upon peers than are females. And females seem to be more dependent on literature and media than males. This information can be helpful to parents as they attempt to balance the effect of peers and the media.

Thornburg defines early adolescence as ages 10 to 15. His research shows that 99 percent of all sexual information is learned during these early adolescent years. More specifically, ages 12 and 13, approximately grades 7 and 8, are the peak ages at which sexual concepts are learned. Of course, any parent of a junior high student could probably have related the same information without doing any research. Junior high is a very stressful and difficult time for parents, and it's not easy

---

Parents must evaluate their children's peers and their influence, since peers obviously play a major role in a child's sex education.

---

on the kids either. Some areas of sex education are particularly appropriate for junior high adolescents, and we will be discussing these in a later chapter.

The last part of Thornburg's article is related to the accuracy of initial sexual information. Twelve topics were evaluated as being highly accurate, accurate, distorted or highly distorted. Information regarding several items was ranked as highly accurate: abortion, conception, intercourse, menstruation and venereal disease. The two subjects covered by the most reliable sources of information were conception and menstruation. In both cases the mother was the primary contributor. The areas which seem in need of more accurate information were: contraception, ejaculation, seminal emissions, homosexuality and masturbation.

This should give you a good starting point in your attempt to provide accurate sexual facts and to correct false and incorrect information your children may have.

Thornburg's work on early adolescence reaches several conclusions which may provide beneficial information for parents. First, adolescents learn most information about sexual behavior from their peers. This has tremendous implications for parents as they try to teach their children about sex. For example, who are the peers of your children? Are their closest peers male or female? What values do these peers and their families hold? How much time does your child spend with these friends? Parents must evaluate their children's peers and their influence, since peers obviously play a major role in a child's sex education.

A second pertinent conclusion from this article concerns mothers and fathers and their respective roles. According to the data, mothers play an important information giving role in the areas of conception, intercourse and menstruation. Fathers, regrettably, play virtually no role in providing sex information. Christian fathers have a God-given responsibility for leadership in the home. That responsibility means we must take an active role in our sons' and daughters' sex education.

Thornburg's work also concludes that females tend to seek out more reliable sources of information than do males. This phenomenon is in part explained by the "macho" image males are frequently taught to project. Boys do not cry; they do not appear to be weak, and they do not admit a lack of knowledge or ask questions. In addition, boys in early adolescence generally talk less about feelings and emotions than do girls of the same age. Whatever the reason, it is important for parents of boys to know that their sons are less likely than girls would be to seek out reliable sources of sexual information.

Lastly, this work concludes that, while overall accuracy seems to be increasing, there are still some key areas which seem to be subject to highly inaccurate information. These areas are contraception, homosexuality and masturbation. These areas of inaccuracy are centered on some of the most controversial aspects of human sexuality, but as Christian parents, we must be sure that our children are taught God's principles in *all* areas of sexuality.

Thornburg closes his article by saying:
Regardless of the findings of this and other studies about teenage sexual understanding, they typical-

ly have learned only partial concepts and basically stand in need of increased or more complete
information about human sexual behavior. Many
are still quite naive, and the risk of naivety among
many adolescents is too high for responsible
adults to ignore.[2]

Media Influence

Now, let's conduct an experiment. If you have teenagers
between the ages of 13 and 15 answer the following questions:

1. How often do you yell at the top of your lungs, "Turn off
   that TV and go do your homework"?
2. Do you have to remind your teens gently to "turn down
   the stereo or radio?"
3. Do you feel like a chauffeur for the local movie theater,
   especially in the summer?
4. Have you read *Seventeen* magazine lately?
5. Are any of the station selection knobs on your car radio set
   on your stations?

A Junior Achievement report reveals that
media (TV, radio, movies) ranks third,
behind peers and parents, in influencing
the values and behavior of teens.

I have two teenage children—a daughter, 18, and a son, 14.
My answers to the above questions, in order, are: 600, yes, yes,
yes, no. It should come as no shock to parents of teens and preteens that the media has a tremendous effect on our children.
This is true especially with regard to sexual information.

The research I mentioned from the *Journal of Early Adolescence* clearly shows an increasing trend toward media influence
as a prime source of sexual information for children of all ages.
A Junior Achievement report reveals that media (TV, radio,
movies) ranks third, behind peers and parents, in influencing
the values and behavior of teens. This represents a dramatic
shift since 1960 when media ranked eighth behind such factors

as teachers, relatives and religious leaders.[3] Now before you are tempted to think that such a survey would be inaccurate for religious church kids, listen to this information from *Five Cries of Parents:*

> Our study of adolescents shows a strong relationship between exposure to mass media and the following: hedonism (seeing pleasure as the highest goal); use of drugs and alcohol; sexual arousing activity; and the rejection of traditional moral beliefs.[4]

Merton P. Strommen is a Lutheran clergyman as well as a noted research psychologist. He is the founder of Search Institute, an organization which has conducted many major research projects and published several books. The material quoted refers to a survey of over 8,000 adolescents, all of whom were from religious, church attending homes. Mass media is clearly influencing our children, especially with regard to sexual information.

The *Journal of Communication* reported that television portrays six times more extramarital sex than sex between spouses. Ninety-four percent of the sexual encounters on soap operas are between people not married to each other. One research study estimates that the average person views approximately 9,230 sex acts, or implied sex acts, a year on television. Of that sexual activity, 81 percent is outside the commitment of marriage. This means that if the average young person, watching ten years of television from age 8 to 18, watched 93,000 scenes of suggested sexual intercourse, 72,900 of these scenes would have been pre- or extramarital.[5]

Tony Campolo, noted Christian lecturer and author, states that "television must be cited as a major factor contributing to the difficulty of modern parenting. This isn't surprising when we consider the fact that the average child watches five hours of television a day. Television dominates the consciousness of young people."[6] As parents we are aware of the negative effects of television, and we know that today's advertisers use sex to sell everything from toothpaste to cars. Equally alarming is the fact that now most American homes have cable television and children can have unrestricted viewing of R-rated movies.

If you are the parent of a teenager you no doubt have been subjected to a marathon of music. Adolescents love music. From grades 7 through 12 kids listen to an average of 10,500 hours of rock music. The total amount of time spent in school over a period of twelve years is just 500 hours more than the time spent listening to rock music.[7] There can be no doubt that the mass media has a profound influence on our children's sex education. It is, and will continue to be, one of the primary sources of sexual information and attitudes for children, and is often at odds with the values Christian parents would like to communicate to their children. The question is, how do we neutralize this massive media influence on our children?

What's a Parent to Do?

Neutralizing media influence is not an easy battle. I have fought and failed many times. My fourteen-year-old-son is a battle-scarred veteran of this combat. Every time I formulate a new tactic, he devises a scheme to defeat my strategy. His latest argument was based on his need for relaxation before encountering the dreaded nighttime nemesis called homework. He very carefully and logically explained that a few hours of television would provide him with the relaxation required to tackle his very draining homework assignment. I did manage to win this battle, but I'm not sure who's winning the war! In a more serious vein, let me suggest a few ways that parents might neutralize media influence.

Parents should regulate both the quantity and quality of media exposure. We need to set realistic guidelines governing TV, movies and printed material. The key word here is realistic. Obviously in today's society, children are going to be exposed to the media. It would be unrealistic to try to stop all exposure to the media, especially TV. As parents, however, we need to regulate this exposure. I have found that many parents concentrate their regulation on the quality of the program but are not concerned about the amount of time their children spend exposed to the programs. It is necessary to limit the amount of time spent watching television for at least two reasons. First, much of the damaging influence of television comes from the commercials. These commercials often promote promiscuous sexual attitudes, to say nothing of the blatant materialism they portray. In addition, spending hours in front of a television promotes poor stewardship in children. As Christians we are to be good stewards of all that God has given us. One of his most precious gifts is our time. Consistent, realistic regulation of both quality and quantity of television viewing should be one of our goals.

A positive strategy you can employ is to use exposure to the media (especially television and music) as opportunities to talk to your children. Sex education is an everyday on-going process and part of the process involves taking advantage of our opportunities. Watching TV and listening to music with our children and then discussing the values and issues we have encountered provides an excellent opportunity to teach many lessons to our children. By asking questions during a program we can determine their level of understanding. Viewing TV together is an excellent nonthreatening way to discuss many delicate topics, especially sexual matters.

Another strategy is to be creative in providing alternatives to the media. Encourage reading, conversation, outdoor exercise, and many other activities. Also look for good media programming and encourage your kids to view it in place of questionable material. In the area of music, good, contemporary Christian music of all types provides an excellent alternative to traditional rock music. Several years ago when my youth group would travel out of town for an event such as a mission trip, camp or retreat, most of the music played was non-Christian rock music. Today, thanks to local concerts, and personal friendships with Christian musicians, at least 80 percent of the music played on our youth trips is contemporary Christian music. Providing alternatives requires work, planning and creativity on the part of parents, but the benefits derived from wholesome alternatives make the effort worthwhile.

One of the best ways to replace our children's exposure to the media is to give them our time. Consider this statistic: 53 percent of teenagers report spending less than 30 minutes a day with their fathers, and 43 percent of teenagers report spending less than 30 minutes a day with their mothers.[8] Parents often use TV to get their children out of their way. They are too busy so they let TV baby-sit. We cannot positively influence the sexual development of our children or neutralize media influence if we do not spend time with them. Furthermore, simply turning off the TV will do nothing to teach our values to our children. It may stop them from being exposed to negative, unchristian values, but it will not teach them godly values. This requires spending time with them; for without a positive relationship it is impossible to have a positive influence on a young person's sexuality. The most effective way to counteract the negative influence of the media then, is to replace the exposure to the media with time spent with you. Fortunately, given the choice, most children, especially preadolescents, will choose to spend time with a parent rather than watching TV.

For Further Thought

1. What are the sources of my children's sexual information?
2. Am I a source of sexual information for my children?
3. Who are my children's closest friends (peers)? What are the values of these friends? How much time does my child spend with these friends?
4. How do I feel about contraception, homosexuality and masturbation?
5. What are my children's favorite television programs and movies?
6. What are my children's favorite musical groups? What are these groups' lyrics promoting?
7. What specific plans have I made to neutralize the effects of the media on my children?

Chapter 3

HEY, MOM, CAN I ASK YOU SOMETHING? (BECOMING ASKABLE)

My wife had volunteered our services. It was all settled, we were to have our four-year-old nephew to stay for three glorious days. Jordan loves his Uncle Scott (that's me), and he jumped at the chance to stay at our house for three days. He feels totally comfortable and at ease around our family.

Included in Jordan's three-day stay was a Sunday, and we took Jordan to Sunday School and worship services. During the sermon as our minister was attempting to emphasize a particular point, he shouted loudly and hit the pulpit. An uncomfortable congregational silence followed. Then Jordan turned to me, gestured toward the pulpit with his hand and shouted, "What's he mad about?"

Everyone, including the minister, heard Jordan's question. I was embarrassed and wanted to hide under a pew. Jordan, however, was totally innocent and was genuinely puzzled by the minister's behavior. He felt totally comfortable asking me this question. He trusted his Uncle Scott to provide an honest answer to his inquiry. I was a primary source of information for him.

In the last chapter we pointed out that parents should be more active as primary sources of information for their children. Most parents agree that they should be their child's primary source of information. The key issue then becomes, how do we effectively communicate with our children? In other words, are we askable parents? Do our children, like Jordan, feel free to approach and ask us questions? And, if not, how can we become askable and approachable?

Becoming askable is very important because when parents are not askable, young people invariably get their sex information—often misinformation—from other sources, especially friends. A tremendous amount of sex education occurs in the lunchroom, the locker room, the bathroom, through graffiti, pornography, sex jokes and the boasts and bravado of some of the young people presumed to be sexually active. Young people also receive a great deal of sexual information from movies and television, most of it of a sensationalistic and distorted nature. Children need their parents' rational perspective to help counterbalance the distorted images all around them.[1]

Young people not only need but desire sincere communication with their parents. To provide this communication is important because there is evidence that communication about sexual matters postpones sexual activity. According to several studies, children who do talk with their parents about sex behave more responsibly; that is, they tend to postpone sexual relationships.[2] Communication with your children about sexual matters increases the likelihood that they will not engage in premarital sex.

Effective communication with our children is very important. It is equally important that we begin early to communicate with our children. Parents who rarely communicate with their children when they are very young have the most difficulty talking with their children when they are teenagers. Communication about sex is not something to be limited to a single talk or an occasional talk at significant developmental stages in a child's life. It should be an ongoing process. Becoming an askable parent starts long before the child goes to school. The parents who have discussed sexuality openly with their child can expect the teenager to show confidence later.[3]

Are You an Askable Parent?

If you wish to take the major responsibility for your children's sex education, you will almost certainly have to deal with a variety of questions and behavior, some of which may catch you by surprise or come at inopportune moments. You can also expect, on occasions to be embarrassed by questions much like my nephew, Jordan's. Conscientious parents are concerned about doing the "right" thing when, for example, a child asks a specific question about birth, or finds a magazine with photographs of naked people, or "plays doctor" with other children. But many people are somewhat uncomfortable about these and other aspects of sexual curiosity. This is largely because their own parents did not provide them with effective models for dealing with such things.[4]

By now you are perhaps thinking, "How do I know if I'm an askable parent?" Here is an exercise to help you determine your own "askability." Relax, this is not a test, because there are no right or wrong answers, just your own honest responses. As a parent of two teenagers, and a youth minister of many years, I can assure you these situations and statements are very typical and these, or similar comments, will occur at some point in the lives of most families.

An Askable Parent Quiz[5]

As a parent, you want your answers to be both factual and age-appropriate. The more comfortable you feel in providing adequate answers, the more askable you will be. To test yourself on this score, consider the following situations that are typical of those most parents will face at one time or another. Circle the letter by the response that you think is best. At the end of the quiz I'll give my opinion about the best answer to each question, although the absolutely "right" answer depends on the dynamics of the relationship between you and your child.

1. Your four-year-old asks, "Where do babies come from?" What do you say?
   a. "When you get older, I'll tell you all about it."
   b. "When a Mommy and a Daddy want a baby, and they love each other, they just have one."
   c. "God made a special place in Mommy's body where babies can grow."

2. Ten-year-old Doug comes home from the playground and asks his father what a rubber is. What does Doug's father say?
   a. "It's nothing that you should be concerned about at your age."
   b. "It's something used to keep the woman from getting pregnant."
   c. "It's something a man puts on his penis to keep the sperm from coming out during sex. It keeps the woman from getting pregnant. Rubbers also help prevent sexual diseases."
   d. "Why do you want to know? Where did you find out about it?"

3. Your six-year old asks, "Why do you and Daddy close the door when you go to sleep." What do you answer?
   a. "Sometimes we want to be really loving together, and we just like to be alone."
   b. "That's not really your business, dear."
   c. "We just don't want to be disturbed."
   d. "If you ever come in when that door is closed, you'll be sorry!"

4. Nine-year-old Ted asks his mother, "What are homosexuals?" What should mother say?

a. "They're people who are attracted to their same sex instead of the opposite sex."

b. "They're very sick people, and you'll become one if you don't stop playing with girls so much."

c. "They're people who are attracted to their same sex the way your Dad and I are attracted to each other. The Bible says it's wrong to act on that kind of feeling."

d. "They're people who aren't normal, and the less said about them the better."

5. Your 13-year-old daughter asks if a male could ever urinate in the vagina during intercourse. What do you say?

a. You tell her you don't really know, and that she should ask her health teacher.

b. If you know, you tell her straight out that the sexual function prevents the urinary function. If you don't know, you say you aren't sure, but that you'll help her find out the answer.

c. You laugh and say, "That's ridiculous!"

d. You try to hide your embarrassment and quickly change the subject.

6. Eight-year-old Kenny says, "I saw Tom and Sue kissing with their mouths open, and Joey calls that 'yukky kissing,'" and asks, "Why is it yukky?" What do you answer.

a. "One name for it is 'French kissing.' A lot of people really in love don't find it yukky...but it sure could spread germs, couldn't it?"

b. "It's totally disgusting, and I don't want to hear you talk about it."

c. "It's a kind of kissing reserved for grownups."

7. Your nine-year-old comes home from school and asks you the meaning of a couple of obscene words he saw painted on the wall. How do you respond?

a. "I don't know."

b. "They're bad words for sex and I don't ever want you to say them."

    c. "They're not polite words, and we don't use them in this house."

    d. "They're sex words people sometimes use when they're angry, or when they want to put someone down. The Bible says our speech ought to be pure, not dirty."

8. Your four-year-old comes to you and asks, "What's the difference between boys and girls?" What do you say?

    a. "Oh, you know...."

    b. "God made girls' and boys' bodies different, so girls could be mommies and boys could be daddies. Girls have a vagina and boys have a penis."

    c. "Girls cook and clean and boys go to work when they grow up."

9. Your eight-year-old daughter asks whether it hurts to have a baby. What do you say?

    a. "Yes, it hurts for a while, but the doctor shows you special exercises and ways to breathe that help. And most women think it's worth it, since a baby is one of God's most precious gifts."

    b. "You're too young to worry about that, dear."

    c. "No, no—it's a wonderful experience."

10. You discover that your four-year-old son has been "playing doctor" with your neighbor's five-year-old daughter—without clothes, of course. What do you do?

    a. Say to your son, "Young man, around here we wear clothes when we play, don't we?" After the two are dressed and his friend has gone home, say, "Let's talk about what you learned when you were playing doctor."

    b. Send the other child home with an "Are-you-going-to-get-it!", then punish your child.

    c. Say to both children, "This is not a nice thing to do. Do you want me to say you can't ever play together?"

11. Mother's five-year-old son asks, "Why do you have big breasts and I don't?" What should she say?

a. "Go ask your father."
b. "Just because I'm a girl and you're a boy."
c. "Because when mommies have babies they may want to feed them milk from their breasts. That's the way God made us."
12. What do you tell a six-year-old who asks, "How do babies get inside a mommy's stomach?"
a. "You'll learn soon enough. Have you practiced your letters today?"
b. "God has made a man so he can plant sperm—or seed—in his wife's body through his penis, in a very loving way. The seed finds its way into the mommy's womb—not her stomach—where it looks for the mommy's egg. If it finds one, they come together, making a baby! It grows until it's ready to be born through the woman's vagina. Isn't that a wonderful plan?"
c. "By a man and woman loving each other."

Well, now—let's see how your answers compare with my opinion of the best answer to these questions. Remember, the "right" answer depends upon the situation and your relationship with your children. As parents our goal is to become approachable and askable. Therefore, our attitude as we answer these questions becomes almost as important as the facts themselves. We should calmly relate the facts in a loving manner. We should also take advantage of every opportunity to present sexual information in a moral context.

1. "Where do babies come from?" is a typical question often asked by children four or five years old. In my opinion "c" accurately answers the question and communicates openness and askability. This response factually answers the question without relating complicated details that could not be understood by a typical four-year-old. It also introduces God as a part of the process. Notice that this answer did not say that a baby is in Mommy's tummy, but in a "special place" for babies to grow. Babies do not grow in tummies, and even

four-year-olds need accurate, age-appropriate information. Answer "b" responds vaguely to the question and would be confusing to a four-year-old. Answer "a" is the least desirable answer because it discourages natural curiosity and openness. By asking questions, children generally indicate their desire for information. Most children will not ask complicated questions beyond their ability to understand the answers. Becoming an askable parent means answering questions when they are asked.

2. Unfortunately, in today's world most 10-year-olds probably know something about condoms. They may lack accurate and appropriate information, but most will have some knowledge of them. The question may have been asked not only to gain additional information but also to test the father's openness and askability. Answers "a" and "d" are both objectionable because they indicate disapproval, and because they make no attempt to answer the question. Telling children they should not be concerned about an issue hinders communication and decreases the likelihood of future questions. Response "b" accurately answers the question, but in my opinion does not provide enough information. Answer "c" goes further and gives additional pertinent knowledge, so I believe it best answers the question. "C" also introduces the subject of sexual diseases. While most 10-year-olds are not ready for in-depth discussions on sexually transmitted diseases, introducing the subject can lead to such discussions in the future.

3. Closing the bedroom door may appear to contradict parental goals of openness and approachability, but a proper explanation can satisfy inquisitive minds without indicating to children that your mind is closed. The worst answer in this foursome is "d." Threatening or overreacting to genuine childhood curiosity squelches communication and guarantees that children will quickly learn that their parents are not askable. Responses "b" and "c" are technically accurate because there are times when parental affairs are not the children's business, and when you have a right not to be disturbed. But

please remember that our goal is becoming askable in order to effectively teach our children about sex. Answer "a" subtly suggests parental lovemaking, without unduly revealing more than a six-year-old can comprehend. Its tone also promote openness.

4. Questions regarding homosexuality frighten most Christian parents. Consequently, we may be tempted to answer questions dealing with this subject less openly and honestly. But inquiring children will ask about homosexuality. And if they sense a reluctance to discuss this or any subject, our approachability will suffer. We must try to remain composed and unruffled even when fielding questions that shock and startle us. Responses "b" and "d" reflect a lack of composure. Also, "d" discourages any dialogue on the subject. Such a reaction might prompt children to seek their information from non-Christian sources. Response "b" creates unnecessary alarm and fear in children. Answer "a," much like several of the answers to other questions, does not furnish enough information. When parents give short, abrupt answers, they can miss opportunities to teach and reinforce moral and biblical lessons. The best answer, "c," supplies factual data an moral teaching, without producing fear in the child. Additionally, "c," leaves the impression that you are open to discussing the subject further if the child wishes.

5. This question accurately identifies a common fact about early adolescents' sexual understanding. While they understand certain aspects of human sexuality, they often have many other misconceptions and misunderstandings. It's not uncommon for them to be confused about bodily functions and the physical aspects of sexual intercourse. The two worst responses to this question are "c" and "d," since they will probably guarantee that future questions will not be directed to the parent. Answer "c" belittles and laughs at the adolescent. No one likes to be ridiculed, so this answer would also severely curtail future communication. While not as bad as "c," answer "d" would also diminish the probability of future conversations, especially regarding sexual matters. If possible,

parents need to project an attitude of happiness and fulfillment with regard to their own sexuality and marital sexual
relationship. Such an attitude lived and modeled before our
children will create an atmosphere in which wholesome,
godly, sex education can be both taught and "caught."

Answer "a" is adequate, but does not go far enough and
hints at reluctance to discuss sexual matters. Answer "b," on
the other hand, straightforwardly provides the facts if they are
known. And if not, it admits a lack of knowledge, and promises to help the adolescent find the answer. Teenagers appreciate parents who readily admit that they do not have all the
answers, and who willingly help in the search for correct
information.

6. Eight-year-old boys probably find all kissing "yukky."
But as we all know, that will rapidly change. Response "a" best
answers Kenny's question. It furnishes sufficient data without
giving more information than an eight-year-old needs or
desires. Responses "b" and "c" are somewhat dishonest,
because French kissing is neither totally disgusting nor
reserved exclusively for grown-ups. Of course, as children
approach adolescence certain warnings regarding French kissing should be provided.

7. Inevitably, our children will come into contact with
filthy and obscene words. Such situations should be viewed as
teachable moments which provide excellent opportunities to
teach about the importance of pure speech. Answer "a" would
be harmful because of its dishonesty. Answer "b" correctly
identifies the words as bad, but it does not utilize the teachable opportunity and thus fails to move toward the goal of
providing godly sex education. Answer "c" makes no attempt
to explain why the words are not polite or why they should
not be used. Children need and deserve such explanations in
order to learn. Answer "d" directly and frankly labels the
words as sex words and further explains why and how they
are used. It also takes advantage of the teachable moment to
explain why the words are inappropriate and to portray
wholesome sexuality in a marital relationship.

8. At about four or five years of age, children begin to recognize and become curious about anatomical differences. This curiosity will inevitably lead to many questions relating to the physical differences between boys and girls. Response "a" evades the question and communicates an unwillingness to be bothered by questions. The probable effect of such evasiveness will be that in the future questions will not be asked. Not only does answer "c" seem flippant and frivolous, but it also subtly promotes sexism. Answer "b" correctly assumes that by "differences" most four-year-olds are referring to physical differences. These differences are simply explained, using age-appropriate and correct terminology. Also, God receives the credit for these differences. By saying that God created these body parts, children are being taught that their entire body is godly and wholesome—a very important lesson for a four-year-old.

9. Preadolescent girls frequently ask questions about birth. They know that this experience will eventually occur in their life, and they are somewhat apprehensive. I feel that answer "b" patronizes even an eight-year-old. It also makes no attempt to answer the question. Dishonesty makes answer "c" totally undesirable. Above all, children need honest, accurate information, and if you fail to furnish correct information they will eventually seek the facts elsewhere. Answer "a" acknowledges that childbirth involves pain, while at the same time explaining specific measures that make the pain bearable. The honesty and correctness of this answer addresses an eight-year-old girl's apprehension and fear. In the future this young lady will feel free to ask additional questions because by being truthful and honest her parents have created an atmosphere of trust and openness.

10. "Playing doctor" or engaging in some such form of physical exploration naturally occurs around ages four or five. Such play indicates a normal curiosity regarding anatomical differences and does not imply sexual perversion or homosexuality. Response "c" accuses and threatens in a very inappropriate manner. These children were satisfying a natural child-

hood curiosity, not being immoral or mean. An accusation of this nature would communicate to a young child that certain body parts are dirty or unclean. In order for healthy sexual adjustment to occur, children need to be taught that God created all of their body, including their genitals. By following upon the threat of response "b," a parent would be punishing a child for a natural curiosity. This response also indicates a level of anger on the parents part that would not be understood by the child. Response "b" also provides no explanation for the anger and furnishes no teaching to the child. Obviously, response "a" best deals with this normal, yet delicate situation. This response informs the child that in polite society people stay dressed. But it also takes advantage of a teachable opportunity in a non-threatening and calm manner. Effective sex education utilizes such moments to provide facts and information at precisely the time of greatest awareness and need.

11. Not only are five-year-olds interested in anatomical differences; in all areas of life they want to know, "Why?" Parents need to keep in mind that by asking such questions children are not obsessed with sexual thoughts; they are simply asking logical questions in their attempt to learn. We should answer sexual questions as matter of factly as we would answer questions on any subject. Answer "a" evades the question and subtly communicates that boys should talk to fathers and daughters to mothers. Both parents must be involved in the sex education of their children. Answer "b": simply states a known fact and does not really answer the child's question. This young man knows that boys and girls have different bodies; his real question relates to the function of female breasts. By answering with the information contained in "c," parents communicate their understanding of the real question. This answer explains the function of female breasts, and attributes it all to God's plan.

12. However children phrase the question, "How do babies get inside of a mommy's tummy?" it often produces fear and anxiety in parents. Perhaps this is true because we realize that

once this question has been asked the process of sex education has reached the point of no return. Also, any honest attempt to answer the question forces us to discuss sexual intercourse. Of course, the discussion must be age-appropriate, but it must be addressed. Response "a" totally dodges the question and attempts to change the subject. If they are repeatedly confronted with such parental avoidance, children will stop asking questions and will simply turn elsewhere for information. Answer "c" is unacceptable for the same reason. Answer "b" lovingly and in an age-appropriate manner explains conception to a six-year-old. This answer corrects misunderstandings and furnishes uncomplicated informa-

---

Many children are crying out for a real conversation with a parent, a dialogue which involves not only the exchange of thoughts, but also of feelings.

---

tion. It also correctly identifies and names body parts using the appropriate terms. Correct terminology helps avoid myths and misconceptions as children learn about sex. When simple age-appropriate sexual information is communicated in a calm, loving manner, childhood curiosity is satisfied and facts are easily accepted.

The best answers to the above questions illustrate how parents can respond adequately to questions related to sex and sexual matters. When answering sexual questions, just remember to:

- furnish the information requested
- use age-appropriate language and concepts
- look for the implied or "real" question
- use proper terms, not slang or cute words
- provide information that leads to the next logical question.

Many of the answers and concepts referred to in this quiz will be discussed in detail in the remaining pages of this book.

Communicating with Our Children

In one of Josh McDowell's books he relates this comment from a teenage boy:

> "Do you know what I am? I'm a comma. Whenever I talk to my dad, he stops talking and makes a comma. Then when I stop talking, he starts right up again as if I didn't say anything. I'm just a comma in the middle of his speeches."[6]

Many children feel exactly like this teenage boy. They are crying out for a real conversation with a parent, a dialogue which involves not only the exchange of thoughts, but also of feelings. They also want a talk that involves both listeners and a talkers. Here are a few principles which can help us communicate effectively with our children. This list is neither unique nor all-inclusive. It is simply several suggestions that will hopefully make communication with your children easier and more efficient.

1. *Remember that rules without relationships lead to rebellion.* Long before the rules are imposed, there needs to be a relationship. In my ministry I repeatedly witness a sad situation. A child does something morally or ethically wrong and the parent approaches me and says, "How could this happen? We've clearly taught our child the biblical principles and rules governing that kind of behavior." In many, but not all, of these incidents the parents have emphasized rules over relationships. Sadly, parents can formulate many rules and regulations designed to produce compliant, well-behaved children, but if they do not invest heavily in relationships with their children, all of these rules will produce rebellion instead of response.

2. *Spend time with your children in their world.* As we stated earlier parents need to spend time doing things with their children. Perhaps go out to eat, just you and one child. Other activities could include shopping, hunting, walking or anything else you both enjoy. These unstressed,

low-key times together can help parents promote good, open communication on the feeling level. During this time with your child, constantly try to see things from your child's viewpoint. Make an attempt to see their adolescent world, because it truly is different from your adult world.

3. *Show trust in the comments or statements of your child.* Too many children, especially teenagers, say that living in their house is like serving a jail sentence, or being continually on trial. They feel as though they are continually looked upon as guilty and have to prove their innocence. Many parents do look upon their children as guilty until proven innocent, instead of innocent until proven guilty. But we must be willing to trust, even though our trust may be violated at times. If your child has violated your trust, you might try saying something like this: "Yes, I trust you to use your own best judgment, but I know from my own experience that one person's best judgment may not include quite enough important facts or knowledge to be completely dependable. And sometimes it may need buttressing with some help from others— even parents. If it's important to you that we trust you to use your best judgment, will you trust us to use our best judgment in the questions we raise and the suggestions we make?"[7] Parents, it is essential that you trust your child as much as possible.

4. *Be encouraging, positive, and noncritical with your children.* All humans need and respond to encouragement. Children especially need their parents to be positive and encouraging. Encouragement can make all the difference in the world. Look at the example of the apostle Paul. After his conversion he was rejected by the Christians in Jerusalem because they were afraid of him (Acts 9). He was shuffled off to Tarsus and might have died there had not Barnabas looked him up and asked for his help (Acts 11). And from that point on, Barnabas, whose name means Son of Encouragement, encouraged Paul, and his

encouragement helped Paul to become a great man of
God. Why is it that, even though we are aware of the positive results encouragement has on our children, we often
seem locked into a pattern of negative criticism toward
them? My 14-year-old son stung me several days ago
with this question: "Dad, do I ever do anything right the
first time?" I said, "Sure you do, Paul." He replied, "Then
why don't you ever tell me?" He was right. As parents we
feel responsible for our children's behavior and morality,
so we criticize, nag and fuss all the time. Please do not
wait until you are stung by your son or daughter. Encourage your children often in positive, noncritical ways.

5. *Check your timing.* In any relationship dialogue will be
enhanced if the timing is right. Love must be your guide
as to when and where you share bad news or discuss a
difficult subject with your teen. For example, never
embarrass your child in front of his peers or in any
crowd. If correction is necessary it will wait until a more
private moment. Parents, make sure your criticism or correction will have a positive, uplifting effect, rather than
be a negative put-down. Choose your time wisely and
never burn bridges.

6. *Never assume.* I am, by nature, a very loud, demonstrative,
excitable and passionate person. I can very quickly
bcome excited and passionate on a great many subjects.
When this happens I usually get very loud and demonstrative. Because of this, many people assume I'm angry,
when in reality I'm just fervent and enthusiastic. My
daughter has always been very calm and laid-back, like
her mother. She has always known how to interpret her
excitable father, and when I would go off like a rocket on
some subject she would simply shrug and just walk away.
She instinctively knew that I was not angry, and especially was not angry with her. My son, on the other hand, is
a very sensitive child and he began at an early age to
have very bad nightmares. We took him to a psychologist
friend who told me that I was the primary cause of my

son's nightmares. Apparently, when I became loud and demonstrative, my son would believe I was angry, and he usually thought I was angry with him. Needless to say, I worked on correcting my behavior in a hurry. But my point is this: I assumed that because my wife and daughter understood the way "daddy was," my son and others also understood. We do our children a grave injustice when we make too many assumptions. All our relationships will become more harmonious and intimate when we stop assuming and start communicating.

7. *Give a little.* Learn the healthy act of compromise. As children grow older they want more freedom and input about the things that affect their lives. Parents need to

---

**Communication is essential to showing love.
Children will not talk to parents about
sex, or anything else, if parents are
not askable and approachable.**

---

understand this and learn the art of compromise.

8. *Follow basic rules for good communication.* Here are some rules that are keys to effective communication in any situation. Some of them are so obvious we tend to overlook them when dealing with our own children. Don't!

- Remember that actions speak louder than words.
- Make your communication as positive as realistically possible.
- Test all your assumptions verbally.
- Recognize that any event may be seen differently from different points of view.
- Do not allow discussions to turn into destructive arguments.
- Be open and honest about your feelings.
- Do not use unfair communication techniques; do not engage in "dirty fighting."
- Realize that the *interpretation* others put on your words

or actions is what is communicated, not necessarily what you *meant* by them.

- Accept all feelings and try to understand them; do not accept all actions, but try to understand them.
- Be tactful, considerate and courteous, and show respect for each family member.
- Do not make excuses and do not fall for excuses.
- Do not nag, yell or whine.
- Learn when to use humor and when to be serious.
- Learn to listen.
- Do not fall into the trap of playing destructive games.

Communication is essential to showing love. Children will not talk to parents about sex, or anything else, if parents are not askable and approachable. Becoming askable and approachable is a lifelong process. It must begin when our children are young and continue through the teen years. Parents must strive constantly to improve their communication skills, because they will never have a major influence on their children's sex education, or any other significant matter, unless and until the children feel comfortable, understood, and at ease discussing all matters with them. You may have all the necessary information regarding any subject, but unless there is a good relationship, your child will never ask for the information.

For Further Thought

1. What is my most frequent method of communicating with my children?
2. Am I afraid to become askable or approachable, and if so, why?
3. How much quality time do I spend with my children each week?
4. What specific traits or characteristics of my children can I encourage?
5. How can I improve my communication with my children?
6. What assumptions about my children do I make?

Chapter 4

BOUNDARIES, GUIDELINES, FENCES, COWS AND KIDS

We have talked about becoming askable—how we can cultivate attitudes that make us approachable. We have talked
about methods of communicating effectively with our children. We have stressed the fact that in order to communicate
with our children it is essential that we have strong relationships with them. Good relationships, however, depend upon
rational, reasonable, firm guidelines and boundaries. The key
to this entire process is BALANCE.

> Balanced growth by the adolescent is best encour-
> aged by the presence of parental guidelines. Just as
> a plant grows the straightest when attached to a
> stake, so a child needs the stability of straight
> guidelines from the parents. Children feel more
> secure when they know the boundaries of the play-

ing field. They will disagree with the boundaries, and in some instances will ask that the boundaries be changed, but they do like boundaries.[1]

Boundaries or guidelines within the family are like fences for cows or skin on the body. They have two purposes: to keep everything in that needs to be in, and to keep everything out that needs to be out. They can also act as a map for children, giving them direction in a society which presents a multitude of options. Giving children guidelines, therefore helps them to make wise decisions.

Parenting Styles—Do I Have to Choose?

Before we discuss how we can set reasonable guidelines and limits, we need to discuss briefly parental discipline styles. They can be divided broadly into three categories.

1. Authoritarian or strict parental style

Christian and secular psychologists describe authoritarian parents as the kind who are usually long on use of the rod and short on use of dialogue. For the authoritarian parent obedience is a virtue, and punishment for willfulness or disobedience is swift. Authoritarian parents insist that the child take their word for what is right, and verbal give-and-take is not encouraged. Authoritarian parents are strong on control, but weak on support, or love. Morton Strommen, in his fine book, *Five Cries of Parents*, quotes several studies that relate to authoritarian or autocratic parents:

> Findings in Study of Generations show that parents who are autocratic in treatment of their children tend also to be law-oriented in their understanding of religion. This means they view Christianity as basically a set of rules and standards that must be obeyed. Such parents find it hard to forgive and hard to admit they are wrong. Their religion tends to be self-centered and self-serving. In comparisons

between groups we found greater family disunity and more distance between parents and youth in the families of overly strict parents than any other group. We found the effect of over control on youth to be lower self-esteem and heightened feelings of self-condemnation. Another frequent outcome is parent-youth conflict, with life in the home becoming an ongoing power struggle. Adolescents raised under autocratic control are more likely to be characterized by the following behaviors: hostility to parents, age prejudice; antisocial activities (for example, lying, fighting, vandalism); feelings of social alienation; rejection of traditional moral standards; an inability to relate well to people.[2]

Authoritarian parents are usually the ones who "provoke their children to anger" (Eph. 6:4, *KJV*).

2. Permissive parental style

Permissive parents are at the opposite end of the scale. They are described as making few demands for obedient behavior, and they usually see themselves as merely resources to be used at the discretion of the child. These parents do not punish and they allow children to run their own lives. They do not make an issue of rules or limits and they shun the use of power to control their children—instead they appeal to reason. Permissive parents are usually strong on support and love but weak on control. Children reared in permissive home environments often feel that their parents really do not care about them. Permissiveness causes teenagers to feel neglected or rejected. Dr. Strommen says of children from permissive homes:

Fewer are likely to go out of their way to help people; fewer are willing to live by the moral standards of their parents (with respect to stealing, lying,

drinking); more are likely to become involved in
hedonistic behavior (use and abuse of alcohol, sex,
drugs); more will seek out movies that are sexually
explicit and erotic.[3]

3. Authoritative parental style
The authoritative parent could be described as someone
who exerts firm control, but who is at the same time willing
to listen. Authoritative parents are inclined to explain their
reasoning and their boundaries. They value both independence and internally disciplined conformity in their children. Authoritative parents are a comfortable mix—taking

> As parents we should strive for
> a reasonable, balanced approach
> to discipline and boundaries.

the strengths of the authoritarian and the permissive parents and combining them into a system that is both high
on support and love and high on control. Children from
authoritative homes usually are better adjusted and more
service oriented. When this parental style is applied, there is
more family closeness and the children are more commit-
ted to a religious faith.

Extremes Can Produce Negative Results
Both extreme styles of parenting (authoritarian and permissive) can produce at least two major problems in children.
First, both approaches may create children with an inability to
interact with and relate to people. The child from the authoritarian home has been taught not to talk back or question, and
just to meet the standards. The permissively raised child has
been taught that he will receive the necessary help to meet
what few standards he wishes to attain. Neither child learns
independence or autonomy. Therefore, both are ill-equipped
to handle most of life's obstacles. The second problem is that
extreme parental discipline styles customarily and typically

produce deviant behavior in children, especially adolescents. This is borne out by all of my research and personal experience in many years of youth ministry. As parents we should strive for a reasonable, balanced approach to discipline and boundaries. We must develop a style that will not "provoke our children to anger", but at the same time will allow us to rear them "in the training and instruction of the Lord" (Eph. 6:4).

Guidelines and Principles for Establishing Practical Limits

My son and I had just had disagreement number 642, but who is counting? Our latest argument concerned his being able to ride in a car alone with a fifteen-year-old. It seems that his friend had received a hardship driver's license and was able to drive at fifteen. Now it seems to me that at age sixteen, the legal age for a license in most states, a teenager is barely mature enough for the awesome task of controlling two tons of steel speeding down a highway at sixty miles per hour. But to trust this tremendous responsibility to a boy newly turned fifteen years old was more than I could imagine. So I refused my son permission to ride with his friend. And, as you may have guessed, my son wanted to discuss the matter!

His first tactic was to attempt a very convincing argument regarding his friend's overall maturity. My counter maneuver was brilliant—I agreed that his friend was indeed as mature as any fifteen-year-old. But my belief was that no fifteen-year-old on this planet was mature enough to drive. My son tenaciously regrouped—he was not yet ready to retreat. He then brought out the time-tested arguments of all teenagers: "Everyone else can ride with him, you don't trust me," and one of my personal favorites, "You're too strict." After several more minutes of discussion, in exasperation I said, "Paul, I love you enough to set limits on your behavior." To which he replied, "If you didn't love me so much, I might have a lot more fun." And with that parting remark he rode off on his bicycle (not in his friend's car).

This incident emphasizes a parental dilemma—how to set

reasonable, realistic boundaries and limits; and once these limits and rules are established, how to enforce them. Setting reasonable boundaries and rules for our children is a day-by-day-job, and there are times when we fail. But as conscientious Christian parents, we can succeed often enough to produce godly children. There are no easy answers or simple formulas, but here are some guidelines, suggestions, and hints that may help you. They are in no particular order of importance, but they are the result of research, personal experience in youth ministry, and parenting two teenagers of my own.

1. *Establish clear standards and rules.* A clear definition of what is acceptable and what is unacceptable behavior is a good starting point. Never assume your child knows what is expected. Children are not mind readers and they need rules explained and demonstrated. If appropriate, discuss the limits with your child before establishing a hard and fast rule. This will help with discipline later on, and can help in establishing a cooperative development of standards. You are not a policeman or a judge. You are a loving, caring parent, who wants to work with your child for his or her good. Never set a limit without giving a good reason. They may not agree, but they will at least understand your reasons.[4] In seeking to determine where your standards will be set, it may be helpful to look at those of older Christian parents. Experienced veterans can be valuable resources as you attempt to avoid mistakes.

2. *Distinguish between biblical absolutes and your personal parental preferences.* God's word has some very specific absolutes. It is unconditionally wrong to steal, lie and commit adultery. But God, in His infinite wisdom, did not make absolutes in all areas of life. Parents must be very careful not to tell their children the Bible clearly supports their own position, unless there are Scriptures that clearly define the issue. We need to tell our children why we believe certain activities are wrong and search the Scriptures with them. But they can read, and if we have been misquoting God, they will ultimately discover our secret.

3. *Know which battles to fight.* Time, strength, and sanity prevent parents from dealing with every potential conflict that arises. Therefore, one of our hardest decisions as parents involves deciding which battles are important enough to fight. As every good general knows, it is possible to win a battle and lose the war, and so we must prioritize and work on those areas which are of greatest importance. Let me illustrate. My eighteen-year-old daughter, Stephanie, has always been a delightful and compliant child. She came into the world that way. Her mother and I had very few major difficulties with her during her growing up years. She was responsible and obedient most of the time. So why does this beautiful, sweet, responsible child insist on living in a garbage dump? I mean, her room is so dirty we are afraid there may be things growing under her bed! Her room looks even worse than her fourteen-year-old brother's. She has no need for a closet and a clothes chest, because all her clothes are on the floor. But my wife and I decided that this was not a battle worth fighting. Stephanie is required to clean before relatives and guests come for a visit, but on an ordinary, day-to-day basis we simply shut the door. And when she runs out of clean clothes she knows how to wash.

4. *Be consistent and fair in defining and applying rules and discipline.* What parent has not heard this cry from their child, especially their teen—"That's not fair!" In my work with teens, I estimate I hear those words at least several million times a year. And yes, I know life itself is not fair, but children need consistently defined rules and punishments. It is disturbing to a child to be confused regarding expectations. Adolescents look for consistent rules in their families, their schools and their communities.

5. *Be flexible and ask for forgiveness when necessary.* As parents we need to be flexible when the situation warrants it, especially when we realize we have made a mistake or a wrong decision. If your child constantly complains about unfairness, you may be wise to check your actions with another

person. If you have been unfair, be flexible and change. Also be godly enough to ask for your child's forgiveness. When we parents admit mistakes we open the way for our children to share with us, and we demonstrate one of God's greatest principles.

6. *Avoid overprotection.* Well-meaning religious parents often make the mistake of being excessively overprotective in the rules and guidelines they establish. These parents continue to do things for their children long after their help has become unnecessary. They break one of the cardinal rules of effective parenting: the parent should not continue to do something for the child that the child can begin to do. Overprotective parents can be very loving, well-meaning people who simply have a difficult time letting go. Overprotective parents project their own insecurity and need for support onto their children. They gain a sense of security by exerting more control over their children's lives, which in turn fosters more dependency on the parent. Through this, dynamic, insecure parents beget insecure children.[5]

The dangers of overprotective parental behavior are many. First, this behavior subtly communicates to the child that his parents feel he is incompetent. David Lewis, a professor at Abilene Christian University, says: "Overworrying produces overprotecting, which produces the message to your child that he is incompetent."[6] A second danger is that overprotectiveness may push children to rebellion, and rebellion can cause serious problems. For example, one of the major reasons for pregnancy in early adolescence (ages 13-15) is rebellion. Finally, children from overprotective environments are usually more susceptible to peer pressure.

Many children allow their parents to wait on them and develop a very demanding attitude, growing angry quickly when things do not automatically go for them the way they wish. They have little personal courage, quickly give in to pressure and give up when faced with a difficult challenge. Deep within overprotected adolescents is an aching feeling of inadequacy and helplessness. They believe that they will never gain the genuine approval of others.[7]

As we suggested earlier when talking about unfairness, when children constantly complain about overprotectiveness on the part of their parents, it may be well for parents to evaluate their behavior in this area. Because the dangers of overprotectiveness are so great, parents should continually monitor their behavior and attitudes.

7. *Use logical consequences to discipline and to teach responsibility.* A logical consequence refers to a natural consequence of an event that is agreed upon beforehand by the parent and the child, and which allows a child to experience the effects of his behavior or unfilled responsibilities in a natural way. When logical consequences are used, the need to nag, remind and gripe is eliminated. Parents simply allow the consequences of a child's action to take hold. For example, if your child chooses to sleep past breakfast time, he will not get to eat until lunch. The child is living with the results of his behavior. If the car is not washed by the appropriate time, it is logical that your son or daughter not be allowed to use the car for a specified time. When logical consequences are applied the focus is on the child's behavior, not on who is right. When teenagers are involved, it is essential that both parent and child together draft the possible consequences of misbehaving or failing to carry out their responsibilities. People often become more responsible when they are helped to recognize the relationship between their behavior and the events which follow. Discipline or punishment that is not connected logically as a consequence to behavior often produces effects that damage the parent-child relationship rather than strengthening it or teaching the child responsibility.

8. *Do not snowplow their road.* Most parents today do a beautiful job of snowplowing the roads for their children. We

think we know what's best for our children, and because we know what's best for them we don't give them enough decision-making responsibility. Then, when our children reach age 18, we throw up our hands and lament the fact that they are irresponsible and cannot make decisions for themselves. As parents, we often don't understand who is to blame for their condition. We are! We snowplow the roads. Let me explain. All too often, we short-circuit the system. We prevent the natural consequences of our children's actions from teaching them valuable lessons. We fix all their messes and failures. We intervene with teachers, employers, coaches and other adults to prevent our children from suffering the consequences of their actions. As a result the lesson they learn is that their parents can remedy any negative consequences of their actions. This produces people who cannot effectively make decisions and accept responsibility for the consequences of these decisions. Within reason we need to allow the consequences of our children's actions to teach them responsibility. In other words, don't short-circuit the system or snowplow the roads. If you say something is going to happen in terms of discipline or consequences, be sure it happens. Do not rob your children of much-needed lessons by repeatedly making empty, vain threats.

9. *Avoid unrealistic expectations.* Often when I counsel kids concerning parent-child conflicts, they cite unrealistic expectations as a major problem. Children, especially teens, feel tremendous pressure because of super high expectations placed on them by parents. Our standards and expectations for our children need to be realistic and attainable. Unrealistic expectations, and the accompanying pressure to achieve, rank high as a major stressor for children.

10. *Accept children where they are.* It is often tough to accept your own child where he is. We don't often have trouble accepting other people's children where they are, but we know how we want *our* children to be, and how we want them to think and act. We don't have to agree with the way our

children are, but it is necessary to communicate that we care for them. If your child's feelings or opinions about anything happen to conflict with yours, try to recognize that he has a right to his feelings. Hear him out and accept him as he is, then go on from there. If he is immature in the way he thinks, your understanding him and accepting him will go a long way toward helping him sort out his feelings.[8]

11. *Listen to your children.* A large part of accepting our children involves listening to them. Nothing builds a relationship faster or better than simply taking the time to be still and quietly listen to our children.

12. *Respect your child's privacy.* One complaint I often hear from adolescents is that parents do not respect their privacy. Children are people, and they should have a right to privacy. Are your children required to knock before entering when your bedroom door is closed? Why should your children not be entitled to the same privacy? Your children are not allowed to listen in on your phone calls, so why should you listen to theirs? Your children are striving for independence, and it is much more desirable for this to take place under the protection of your love and in a safe atmosphere. Of course, there are situations when parents have been given "probable cause" or have a good reason to deny privacy temporarily. That is a different matter. But under ordinary circumstances parents should respect privacy.

13. *Handle problems and conflict in an open, positive way.* Parents cannot rear children in today's world without encountering problems and conflicts. Some of these problems are relatively minor, such as my fourteen-year-old wanting to ride in his fifteen-year-old friend's car. But ultimately parents will be confronted with problems and conflicts of a more serious nature. For example, how should parents handle a child's apparent rejection of family values? Even when hurt, afraid, angry or disappointed, parents cannot panic and allow communication to cease. When children,

especially adolescents, know that their parents are attempting to understand and appreciate their feelings, even when they do not sanction the behavior, a bond of closeness develops between parent and child.

14. *Never embarrass your child—discipline or correct in private.* Children of all ages detest public humiliation and embarrassment. When they are chewed out in front of their friends, it evokes a strong emotional response. At this age they are extremely concerned about the opinion of others, particularly their peers. Your child may need a good old-fashioned chewing out, but have the courtesy to perform the task in private.

15. *Do not use excessive amounts of unrealistic guilt.* I've just lost my daughter! Oh, not for good, but she has recently departed for college. As I said good-bye to her at her dorm, hundreds of memories rushed through my mind: reading *Goodnight Moon* as she dozed on my lap, her first day of school, junior high school, her first date, her first car, her baptism, and many, many others. Leaving her was very traumatic, but I survived. Barely! In the weeks leading up to her departure I attempted to use what I thought was humor to alleviate some of my sadness and loss. I would say to her, "It's okay, just break your parents' hearts and leave home after we've taken care of you for eighteen years! But, don't worry about us, just go ahead and leave." My daughter, Stephanie, took some of this as it was intended—as good, natural humor and a release for her sentimental father. But after awhile she began to feel guilty. And even though it was not my intention, she began to be burdened by this unrealistic guilt. As parents we are sometimes very fearful that our children will not turn out right. This fear causes us to pile guilt on ourselves, and eventually we begin to push some of that guilt onto our children. When guilt is heaped on our children, either purposely or inadvertently, the door to effective communication and input is closed. We can avoid this guilt by spending more time discussing and less time evaluating.

We can also, at times, just keep our mouths closed!

16. *Share yourself and your feelings with your children.* One of the greatest gifts we can give our children is ourselves—not just our money, our support, our car, etc., but the sharing of our thoughts, problems and feelings. This is difficult for most parents because they do not want their children to know that they have problems and fears. But children will receive much comfort, encouragement and strength when they see that their parents are human and that they make mistakes, have problems, and face fears and uncertainties. Parent, share yourself!

17. *Respect your children's choices, and let them fail if necessary.* It is very difficult for most parents to respect their children's

---

Parental limits give children a feeling of being loved and secure and provide a safe environment in which to learn about the real world.

---

choices. As their parents, we are obviously able to make much wiser choices for them! But as children grow into adolescence they need the experience of making their own decisions. The time will come when we will not be constantly at their side, and they will need to function and make responsible choices without our help. How much better to allow our children the opportunity to practice making choices and even to fail while they are under our care and supervision than for them to have their first experience with failure in the outside world! Failure teaches children about the realities of life. There are real responsibilities in the world and kids have to learn how to handle them while they're still in the home. It's the safest place in the world to learn about the realities of life. But, if they don't learn that the real world has teeth and will bite, they will be unprepared to function effectively.

18. *Encourage often.* All people, especially children, need much encouragement. Praise and encourage your children often.

A Final Word and a Letter

All children need structure. They are not ready to be completely out in the world, and they need the firm but reasonable boundaries and guidelines that loving parents provide. Children, especially teenagers, will at times complain and resist rules, but they desperately need and even desire guidelines and restrictions. Parental limits give children a feeling of being loved and secure and provide a safe environment in which to learn about the real world. Hopefully, as parents we can establish firm, reasonable, flexible boundaries that communicate to our children both support and love.

Let me close this chapter with a letter that was written by a young man in his mid-twenties. He wrote this to his father several years ago. This letter very eloquently expresses most of the things I have attempted to convey in the last two chapters. If we, as fathers, receive letters such as this, we will have done our job very well.

Dear Dad,

Well, today is Father's Day, and it seemed like a good time to write this letter. I have intended to write for a couple of years, and now seems appropriate.

I really wanted to let you know what a wonderful father you really are. I know I've said that to you, and I've said thank you, and I love you, and all those things many times before. But I've always wanted to tell you some reasons why, and let you know that when I say those things, they're a lot more than just words.

When I was growing up, especially in high school and college, I would hear my friends and other kids talk about their parents. The way they talked of them was usually not good. They didn't get along with them, they thought they were mean, or weird, or stupid. I felt out of place, because I loved my parents, and thought they were great! In high school and then in college, other kids complained about going on vacations with their parents, or doing things with them; but I enjoyed it! We had fun travelling to Tennessee, or to Florida, or driving across the country.

I realized a lot of the difference between you and those other fathers was the way discipline was handled. When you disciplined me, or wouldn't let me do something I wanted to do (or made me do something I didn't want to do), you always explained the reasons. You always treated me like an intelligent person, who had a right to know the reasons for your actions, rather than just ordering me around. And most of the time, as much as I would have hated to admit it, I agreed with your reasons. Looking back now, I agree with all of them! And I remember one time when you got very angry with me for something that wasn't my fault, you came and apologized later for that. That meant very much to me then and now. I know of very few people who could bring themselves to do that.

One thing that has made me feel the best is the way you have supported me, especially through college and beyond. When I first began seriously considering music as a career, I never heard a negative word from you. It was always encouraging. You would caution me about certain things, certain decisions, but you never criticized my choice. And you even began to listen and study types of music that I know you didn't care for, just so you could offer me advice, and help me out. I didn't (and still don't) know any of my musician friends' parents who did that. There is no way I can ever tell you how much all your concern, advice, time and money has meant to me concerning my music.

I feel very good about myself. I look around at

my family, my accomplishments, and the things I am able to do, and the things I own, and am amazed at how good everything is. And all of it is directly or indirectly because of you and your teaching. One of my most fervent prayers at this time is that I can be the kind of father you are someday to my own kids.

Well, I could go on forever, Dad. I know things are tough there now. I wish I could be there with you, like you helped me through some difficult times. But remember I think of you often, and say a prayer for you.

I love you.

For Further Thought

1. Analyze your parenting style—when are you authoritarian, permissive, authoritative? What patterns do you see emerging? How can you improve your parenting style?
2. Read Eph. 5:1,21; 6:4. How are parents and children to submit to each other? How is your family accomplishing this?
3. Read Heb. 12:5-11. What does this passage tell us about discipline and relationships?
4. What battles do you fight that might be better left unfought?
5. Read Eph. 4:32. When was the last time you asked your child to forgive you?
6. What roads do you snowplow for your children? Devise a simple plan to avoid this in the future.
7. Read Jas. 3:17. This verse is especially relevant to resolving conflicts and working out logical consequences.[9] Are these characteristics present when you resolve conflict and use logical consequences with your children.
8. Can you think of a time when you used unrealistic guilt to motivate your child.

Chapter 5

I DON'T KNOW HOW TO HANDLE A SEX TALK!
(GUIDELINES FOR TALKING ABOUT SEX)

Talking to other people's children is what I do for a living. I'm a youth minister, and I've listened to every question, confession and story you can imagine. Most of the time I can calmly, rationally and factually discuss a wide range of issues and problems with any teen. And I am not easily intimidated by even the most threatening questions. I consider myself a tested veteran of many teenage wars. If all of this is true, then why did I feel so panicked by a single question asked by my son when he was eleven years old? To him it was a simple enough question—"Dad, exactly what is masturbation, and why do people do it?" I had placidly answered very similar questions in many different settings. So why was I so scared? My mind, in computer fashion, was recalling all the volumes of material I had read concerning the do's and don'ts of sex education. Even with all my experience, I still felt unprepared and awkward as I began answering the question. But I suppose my answer was satisfying because, at the conclusion of my answer, he said, "That's what I thought," and calmly walked off.

My experience was similar to that of many parents as they grapple with feelings of fear and uncertainty concerning sexual discussions with their children. Most parents feel woefully inadequate when it comes time to answer specific sexual questions from their children. And this sense of inadequacy is heightened at the prospect of engaging in a sexual talk or discussion. But learning how to talk with our children about sex is very important. Candid discussions with parents contribute

---

**Parents need to equip their children
with the sexual knowledge and
attitudes that can enable them
to make intelligent, godly decisions.**

---

significantly to the development of healthy sexual attitudes. A leading child psychiatrist was asked "What is the best way to prepare maturing boys and girls concerning sexual matters?" The doctor's answer was interesting:

> The best way is an emotionally mature set of parents with a comfortable attitude about sex, and a willingness to answer the child's questions appropriately and honestly. Other approaches (such as school sex education courses) only try to make up for a lack of this and are only second best.[1]

Parents clearly are the key. By talking freely with our children about sex, we train them to be open about sexual matters. We also need to realize that most basic sexual information comes to youngsters from their parents. Children learn their deepest lessons by example and their attitudes toward sex are not so much taught as caught. There are no strict rules or easy formulas to follow here, however. Parents need to equip their children with the sexual knowledge and attitudes that can enable them to make intelligent, godly decisions. To assist you in this formidable task, I have put together some tips and suggestions from several authoritative sources to help you handle sex talks with your children. This information is more general than specific, and is concerned with the "how" of sex talks. The specific "what" information will be discussed later.

One word of caution before we begin. Please do not think that the sex education of your children will be accomplished by a single, or even a few talks or discussions. In order to teach our children effectively about sex, it is necessary to have many such talks in the approximately eighteen years they are at home. What an exciting prospect!

Here's What the Experts Say

1. *Establish the proper climate for sex education.* This involves several factors. First, we must create a loving atmosphere. Parents emit sex education messages to their children from the earliest days of their infancy. The way a baby is spoken to, held, cuddled, picked up, and tucked into bed —all these affect sex education. When these, and other physical contacts are tender and pleasurable, the infant begins to understand how wonderful and comfortable it is to be close to another's body. Through this nonverbal communication the baby finds that relating to other people makes him feel good, happy and accepted. Such a loving atmosphere provides a wonderful setting in which his development as a human being, which includes his sexual development, can take place.

   Another condition of the climate we should aim for in the home is one in which children can see the object lesson of their parents' love for each other. Love is demonstrated in different ways by different families, but the important thing is that love be shown. A child learns a great deal by watching how his mother and father relate to each other. Children need to see devotion, concern, affection and enjoyment of each other's companionship. When children see their parents demonstrate affectionate emotions, it conveys to them the proper meaning of love and respect. And this is a crucial part of sex education.[2]

A third factor helping to create the appropriate climate is for the parent to be relaxed. In the words of Christian broadcaster and author, John Nieder:

> Embarrassment creates anxiety. And anxiety usually cripples communication. If you get uncomfortable talking about sex, you will make your child feel uneasy, and the tension may very well destroy her openness. Next time the topic of sex enters a conversation, make sure you smile...even if your stomach growls, your blood pressure rises, or nausea begins to set in.[3]

Fourthly, parents can create a climate conducive to good sex education by speaking positively about sex. As we have already seen, a primary source of children's sexual information is the media. And the media portrays sex as wonderful and the supreme experience. If we, then, as parents speak about sex only in negative terms, our children will begin to get the idea that to us, sex is evil and ungodly. Our children need sex portrayed as a positive, exciting and wonderful gift from God that is to be enjoyed by married couples. Such a portrayal will place the enjoyable nature of sex within God's perfect plan.

Openness, or "askability," is a fifth requirement for developing a positive climate for sex education. Children should be encouraged from the earliest years to feel at ease in talking with their parents about anything that concerns them. Openness means that we are attempting to understand our children's point of view and are willing to learn and grow with our children. It also means we are prepared to share our thoughts and feelings sincerely with our children. In this atmosphere children will feel free to bring us their questions, doubts and problems without fear of censure and condemnation.

Remember my son's question concerning masturbation? The words I used to answer him were important. But far more important was my reaction to his question. If I had lost my composure and overreacted with a stern warning, he would probably have concluded that I was either ignorant of the facts or I was discouraging his openness. If we want our children to come to us with their sexual questions, we must not discourage their openness and turn them toward less reliable sources of information.

2. *Get an early start.* Your children's world can turn sexual quickly. One day your child may have little curiosity about sex; the next day everyone in the class may be excited over something sexual. Menstruation, masturbation, breasts, erections, dating, kissing, intercourse—all these issues can be stressful to the adolescent encountering them close-up for the first time. If you have prepared your children over several years, they have a good chance of taking such problems in stride. Your early teaching can stand your teens in good stead. But this preparation must be done while they are still receptive to your leadership and before the inevitable periods when they are asserting their independence. There is no precise timetable governing what sexual facts should be furnished at what age. If, however, your child has not started asking sexual questions by age four or five, look for occasions to bring up the subject. Sex education must begin early!

3. *Look for teachable opportunities and take the initiative.* A good teacher does not see her task merely in terms of sitting and waiting until questions are asked. Rather, she tries to stimulate wonder and curiosity so that questions will be asked. A good teacher also knows that learning occurs gradually. As teachers of sex education in the home, we must also keep these things in mind. Some children are very inquisitive and ask questions; other children do not ask questions or stop asking as they grow older. Adolescents are likely to be shy about approaching

parents with specific sexual questions. We are neglecting our responsibilities as parents if we say nothing. It is our responsibility to bring up the subject. Let me give you an example.

Do we allow our children to drift in the hope that someday they will ask about God or find God for themselves? As Christians, we actively share God and His Word with our children. We don't sit back and wait for them to take the initiative and ask us about God. Because of the importance of the issue, and our love for our children, we take the initiative. Why then should sex be a taboo subject? We must take the initiative in discussing sexual matters with our children. And if our children fail to ask questions regarding sexual matters, we as parents must be alert and search for opportunities for teaching.

Opportune moments abound in the daily lives of our children. Suppose your child comes home repeating an off-color joke. You could scold and scream, or you could use the occasion as a teachable moment and teach valuable lessons. You can also find opportunities for teaching while watching TV with your children. During a program about birth control, for example, parents can ask questions, to determine the level of a child's information. If the information is inadequate, then a golden opportunity to teach is available. There are many documentaries, as well as other programs, that feature sexual situations. Teaching opportunities can be discovered in many routine day-to-day situations, such as movies, music, advertisements and books.

Parents should also be alert to teaching opportunities stemming from their children's physical experiences. As young preteens approach puberty the physical changes occurring in their bodies can be used to expand their sexual knowledge. Other natural occurrences in life can provide a good opportunity to discuss sexual issues. A new baby in the family or a litter of kittens can make a wonderful occasion for talking about sex. Sex education opportunities are endless and should be seized. By taking the initiative parents express concern, openness and availability.

4. *Repetition will be necessary.* Sometimes, because of a negative approach by adults, children (especially teenagers) block out sexual information because they are frightened by it. Their earliest memories of parents and other adults discussing sexuality may have led children to believe that sex is dirty, sinful and wrong. These children frequently repress sexual knowledge. Therefore, there may be a need to repeat previously discussed sexual information. In

---

Remember one of our basic axioms: sex education is a gradual process and involves much repetition.

---

doing so, we need to reassure our children that the issues are complex and not easily understood, especially all at once. It is also true that when certain facts are initially discussed, the information is sometimes only partially understood. As the child grows older, the information will have more personal relevance, and will need to be discussed again. Remember one of our basic axioms: sex education is a gradual process and involves much repetition. Parents should not feel they failed to "get through" if a child repeats a question they thought they had explained earlier. The repetition probably means the child is ready for a deeper and broader look at the matter. Gradualness and repetition are the key.

5. *Accept your child's sexuality and earn his trust.* Parents need to communicate to their children that they accept their emerging sexuality and that they will never use against them anything they reveal about their sexuality. Research indicates that adolescents deeply mistrust their parents with regard to sexual feelings. They fear that parents may use this information against them in some way. One

teenager, serving on a panel at a meeting of the American Association of Sex Education, Counselors and Therapists, gave this advice to parents:

> You have to show your kid that he can trust you. You shouldn't throw in a person's face something he did or something he doesn't know. You shouldn't say, "Oh, daddy's little girl shouldn't know that."[4]

Many of the other youngsters on the panel wished that they could talk to their parents about sex, but felt they could not. One panelist said:

> The parent has to make the first move. You have to know that you'll be received, that your parents will accept you.[5]

The feelings of these panelists express both a desire to talk to their parents and also a fear or lack of trust toward parents. In order to remove their fears and establish trust, you must take your children's sexual concerns very seriously. Never make fun of any misinformation they may have, or areas of ignorance. Also, be aware of your child's self-consciousness and embarrassment regarding sexual issues. Under no circumstances should you joke about your child's sexuality. Remember that trust and acceptance are extremely important issues to children, especially adolescents.

6. *Keep it casual and conversational.* Lectures turn kids off and cause them to feel as though they are being spoken at, not to. Informal, casual, spontaneous conversations are more effective in sensitive areas such as sex. One way to keep it casual is to give children time to absorb new information and clarify new ideas. Be brief and leave the door open for additional conversations in the future.

You also need to be prepared for questions to come at odd moments. Children will often initiate conversations regarding sensitive topics when they feel comfortable and at ease, so such conversations may occur during routine family activities.

7. *Calmly and without panic answer your child's questions.* Take your child's questions at face value and answer them factually and calmly. After you have answered the questions, you may find it helpful to ask: "What aroused your interest?" But ask that only after you have factually answered the questions, and have resisted the impulse to jump to conclusions. For example, if your son asks if condoms are effective against venereal diseases, do not assume he is asking because he intends to test the product. Children are very curious and routinely file away all sorts of sexual information they never intend to use. If you make assumptions and jump to conclusions, it may have the effect of scaring off your child and causing him to stop asking questions and seeking advice.

When your child asks a question that is not clear, ask: "In what way?" or "How do you mean?" Follow-up questions like these will help you identify the real issues and prevent you from giving long, tedious explanations that are both unwanted and unnecessary.

8. *Retreat if you encounter resistance.* Parents' efforts to discuss sexual matters can be frustrated by their children. Your children may tell you they already know all they need to know, or they may simply walk away. If this happens, rather than press the topic, or pressure your child, just say, "OK, let's talk about this another time." When we try to force the issue, our children sometimes sense our tension and feel pressured. At this point they become even more reluctant to include us in their sex education. It is never easy to guess the mood of an adolescent, but if you sense problems, trouble or stress, simply wait for these things to pass and look for a more appropriate time. You also need to follow the child's timetable rather than your own. Your child may be worried about a particular stage of puberty, and until that pressing problem is solved, the

youngster will probably not be ready to discuss another sexual topic.

You may also meet resistance if your child senses an invasion of privacy. Teenagers especially have a strong urge to protect their privacy, and they are likely to react defensively if they feel their parents are meddling. Avoid being overly curious and resist the temptation to ask ill-timed personal sexual questions. Such embarrassing questions can cause teenagers to become noncommunicative, evasive and silent. Parents who take intrusive behavior to the maximum limits may also face rebellion from their teens. This rebellion is an attempt on the part of adolescents to pursue their autonomy and to achieve independence. As I have mentioned before, rebellion is one of the primary reasons for pregnancy in early adolescents and a well-timed retreat by parents is sometimes in order.

9. *Use proper terms.* Dr. James Dobson, noted Christian psychologist, once remarked that when it comes to discussing sex, parents usually use "sophisticated" language. He said, "For example, everyone knows that a boy has a 'thing-a-me-jig' and girls have a 'whats-ya-ma-call-it.'"[6] Unfortunately when discussing sex with their children, some parents do not use correct terminology. We do not need to be unreasonably detailed in this regard, nor should we cite every minute technical term and burden tiny children with the vocabulary of a physiology textbook. But correct terminology, commensurate with the child's vocabulary, should be used. When we give the correct names to parts and functions of the body, we aid our children in gaining accurate sexual information. This will also help them to share their feelings about sexuality. The use of correct terminology is important in avoiding inaccurate impressions. For example, a baby does not grow in a mother's tummy. Reproduction is not a function of the stomach or digestive system. Children who have been taught in these inaccurate terms sometimes keep these wrong impressions for years.

Most parents do not use proper terminology because they are embarrassed to do so. One leading psychologist advises parents to say the correct words out loud and listen to themselves. Doing this will help you become less sensitive. You should also refrain from using either euphemisms or obscene language. It is really just as easy to use the correct term for a part of a baby's body as to refer to the part by either a cute or a dirty word. Do not deprive your children of the necessary vocabulary to increase their knowledge and understanding. Correct terminology is a vital part of sex education. As a parent, you will need to know these facts if you are to teach your children correctly. To help you, we have included a glossary of easily understandable terms concerning sexual anatomy and physiology at the end of this book.

10. *Be accurate and dispel myths.* This follows from the previous topic. Use accurate terminology and give accurate information. This includes dispelling myths. The sexual "knowledge" of adolescents often consists largely of myths and folklore...much of it hazardous. Some of the more common myths many young people believe are: females can become pregnant only while menstruating; venereal disease germs can be washed away; only a limited amount of semen can be produced by males over a lifetime (many boys worry that they have used up their supply by masturbating); females cannot get pregnant during their first intercourse; and many, many more. When you squelch myths, however, avoid putting down your child for believing the misinformation. Such treatment can make children feel their concerns are unimportant.

In order for sex talks to be really useful, it is often necessary to be blunt and expose euphemisms. Make no bones about the reality behind a word. For example, abortion is often described as "termination of pregnancy." Let your child know that abortion involves the complete destruction of the fetus. You will be giving the child a reasonable basis for making a decision, and young people appreciate this kind of honesty.

Parents who repeat myths, or who "protect" their children from hard sexual truths, confuse the children and risk discrediting themselves. It is just as much a mistake to distort facts in an attempt to influence your teenager's behavior. Your teen will stop listening to you if you pass on falsehoods, and your subsequent statements, however accurate, will be doubted. Sometimes, even with the best of intentions, parents start out with a credibility gap.[7]

11. *Admit your discomfort in talking about sex and furnish other resources.* Personal discomfort concerning sexual matters prevents some parents from discussing sex with their children. Unfortunately many Christian parents come from restrictive backgrounds that cause them to be more liberated intellectually than emotionally. In other words, you can often say the right thing but you do not feel right saying it. And when this happens, body language, facial expressions and tone of your voice, give you away. This kind of behavior gives children mixed messages and may prompt them to avoid the subject of sex when you are around.

You can overcome some of your difficulties by talking about sex education. Conversations with your spouse, other family members, or a support group, can help you become accustomed to talking about sexual matters. You can also become active in community organizations that deal with sexual issues, such as rape crisis programs, teen pregnancy clinics, or hospital VD clinics. Hopefully, discussing or working with sexual issues will help ease your inhibitions.

No matter how hard they try some parents cannot overcome their inhibitions. If this is your case, tell your children that you are not comfortable talking about sexual matters, and urge them to get instruction and advice from another reliable source. This should really be a last resort as it is much more desirable for you, the parent, to be the primary sex educator of your children. I believe all parents can learn to function in this role to some extent, but if you are not completely satisfied with your abilities, do not ignore your children's sex education. It is too important. Take steps to ensure that your child's sex education will not be neglected.

First, make information available to your children. Many good books and TV programs are available that teach on an appropriate level. Encourage your children's exposure to these media. Second, there are many well-run, realistic sex education courses conducted by schools and churches. Help your youngster sign up for these courses. Third, and most important, encourage your child to find another sensitive adult who can act as a confidant, instructor and advisor. Elizabeth Douvan, a psychologist at the University of Michigan, says:

> Adolescents need contact with satisfied and effective adults, both inside and outside the family. And sometimes the parent/child relationship needs an intervening third person who can mediate and interpret the parties to each other.[8]

12. *Stress the uniqueness of the Christian message and turn to the Scriptures.* From an early age children need to be taught the biblical message concerning sex. Unless your children know the biblical position and the proper context for sex, they may find themselves adrift in a sea of conflicting values. Children need to learn that God loves and cares for them, and that He understands the mysterious stirrings, worries and concerns that occur during adolescence. Children can gain a sense of wonder at God's marvelous creation in their bodies. They can learn that God provides guidelines, gives comfort, and has not abandoned them on a sea of sexual confusion.

In helping our children learn about sex with the gospel

message as a frame of reference, we help them see the truth that God created sex, and the often unrecognized fact that God wants to guide and help us with this powerful and beautiful gift. In her book, *Sex Is a Parent Affair*, Letha Scanzoni explains that according to Scripture, the purpose of sexual activity is fourfold: procreation, recreation, communication and release.

A reading of the Song of Solomon, as well as an understanding of this fourfold purpose of sex, will help young people establish a true picture of the biblical ideal for sex in marriage. God intended married couples to enjoy sex fully. Your healthy attitude toward sex, as well as clear statements and teachings, will help your children understand the proper biblical message concerning sex.

13. *Put sex in proper perspective.* Help your children see that sex is just one part of their lives, and that it is tied to all other feelings. Adolescents, because of their lack of experience, often do not have a realistic perspective on life and tend to be uncertain in their expectations. As an adult and a parent, you have experienced life more fully. Use your experience and wisdom to help your children see that sex is only one part of a successful marriage. It is important, yes, but it is by no means the only consideration. In fact, according to research done by Dr. Sol Gordon (one of the leading experts on sex education in the United States) sex ranks ninth on a list of the ten most important characteristics of a mature marriage:

> Sexual intercourse, as an aspect of our sexuality, is greatly overrated. If some people's public persona were to be believed, however, it would often appear that only nuclear war is a more important issue in our lives.

Here is Dr. Gordon's list of the ten most important characteristics of a mature marriage:
1. Love, caring, and intimacy together.
2. A sense of humor and playfulness.

3. Honest communication and interesting conversation.
4. A passionate source of mission and purpose.
5. Friends together and separately.
6. Commitment to one's own identity and ideals.
7. Tolerance of occasional craziness, irritableness, conflict, error.
8. Acceptance of each other's style.
9. Sexual fulfillment.
10. Sharing household responsibilities.[9]

A Final Word

Talking to children about sex is not easy for parents, so we have discussed the feelings of embarrassment, inadequacy and fear which cause us to approach the topic of sex cautiously. In spite of these misgivings, we can effectively communicate sexual information to our children. To quote Sol Gordon again: "Contrary to modern theory, it simply is not necessary to feel entirely comfortable about sexuality in order to communicate effectively with your children."[10]

These suggestions and tips will hopefully make your sex talks more relaxed and helpful. Remember, however, there are no pat answers. How and when to tell your children about sex is a sensitive issue. In today's world, children are often aware of highly sophisticated sexual facts at an unusually tender age. Even kindergarten children may hear comments that need explaining. But remember, each child is different in his sexual interest, awareness, and comprehension. It is best to think of starting sex education at the birth of your child and making it an ongoing lifetime process

For Further Thought

1. In your home is love openly demonstrated toward each other? How can this be improved?
2. Are you relaxed and positive when talking about sex?
3. List several teaching opportunities that you failed to

recognize at the time. How could you have used these occasions as discussion starters?

4. Do you accept your child's sexuality? Does your child feel this acceptance?

5. Do your children trust you not to misuse your knowledge of their sexual feelings?

6. Anticipate several possible questions that could cause you to panic, and work out answers for these questions.

7. In discussions with your children, which sexual issues, terms, or situations, would cause you the most discomfort? Why?

8. Read Heb. 13:4. See whether you can find four teachings about sex in this verse and think about how you would share them with your teenage son or daughter.

9. How do you think I should have answered my son's question regarding masturbation?

Chapter 6

BABIES, PRESCHOOLERS, AND SEX

I was teaching a parenting class at church and during a question-and-answer period after I had already responded to several questions, a young mother at the back of the room shyly raised her hand and asked very sheepishly, "At what age do you suggest we begin sex education?"

The class laughed and assumed I was joking when I said, "Well, Mrs. Jones you had better hurry up and start because your children are ahead of you; they began at birth."

I quickly explained that I was very serious. Sex education begins at birth! The world of infants is composed almost entirely of the senses. Their world revolves around sounds, smells and temperature. Babies need and desire to be touched. Much nurturing takes place as a mother holds and feeds her child at her breast. Infants very quickly begin learning all about themselves and their world through observation and association. They observe the manner in which they are spoken to, held, hugged, kissed, and then they associate these actions with warmth and security. Since all of these sensual delights are primarily provided by their parents, babies very quickly begin to see themselves exactly the way their parents see them. So parents are influencing and teaching babies from the earliest moments of life. There are many seemingly routine issues surrounding infants and young children that can have a profound effect on their sexual well-being. Sex education truly begins at birth, whether consciously or subconsciously.

Sex Education for Babies (Ages Birth-2 years)

Many things that we learn during infancy stay with us throughout our lives. One of the most important lessons is whether we perceive the world as hostile or friendly. An infant whose needs are regularly met views the world as a friendly, warm place. But an infant whose needs are not regularly met learns to view the world as a scary place where no one can be trusted. The perception of a friendly world is translated into trust and has an effect on how the infant learns to relate to others. As we stated, infants learn trust primarily through touch. The nurturing touch of mother and father, or the lack of it, lets babies know whether it is safe to reach out to others, or better to withdraw. So parents educate their children by the way they hold them, the way they touch the baby's skin, the way they play with the baby; stroking, cuddling and holding him close.[1]

The way you handle your baby and your facial expressions while holding him reflect your opinion of your child. For example, if you react squeamishly or negatively to such normal tasks as changing diarrhea-filled diapers, or medicating messy umbilical cords, what message is your baby receiving? Parents must be extremely careful not to grimace or use body language that communicates disgust during the physical care of their babies. Such behavior can negatively influence an infant with regard to his sexuality.

There are several specific aspects of an infant's physical sex education that are important. Some experiences critically affect an infant's acceptance of his body and his attitude toward body parts and functions. First, as we have already mentioned, parents should avoid reacting with displeasure or disgust toward normal body functions. One day, when our son was a few months old, I returned home after a hard day at the office and found my wife in her underwear, crying in the hallway outside our infant son's room. He had diarrhea and vomited all day long, and he was having so many bowel movements and vomiting spells that he had soiled all of his

---

Parents teach an infant to accept his body by the way they react to his self-discovery; they need to be aware that infants live in a God-given world of sensual delight.

---

mother's clothes. Every time she went in to change him, he would ruin another layer of clothing. It was very quickly apparent that mother was out of clothes and patience. Now my wife, Linda, had the good judgment not to react in displeasure in our son's presence. She saved the disapproval, disgust and frustration for me! But suppose she had reacted negatively in his presence. Suppose she had yelled at him, or simply cried from frustration. How would an infant understand such actions? He would probably be completely confused at this response to his perfectly natural body functions. Since the excretory and sexual organs are in such close proximity, it is difficult for an infant to distinguish between them. Therefore, when parents react with displeasure or seeming disapproval, the baby is learning that certain parts of his body are distasteful or even shameful. My wife's experience that day many years ago was not a pleasurable one, but it is vitally important that parents learn to attend to normal body functions with grace and dignity. If a child grows up believing part of his body is shameful it can adversely affect his sexuality at a later date.

Parents also teach an infant to accept his body by the way

they react to his self-discovery. Have you ever witnessed parents, grandparents and other excited relatives gather around an infant's bed and watch him identify or play with his ears, nose, or feet? They all respond as if he is the most intelligent baby in the world. Each time he correctly identifies a body part he is praised and affirmed. That is, until the little darling reaches for and discovers his genitals! Everyone starts acting very embarrassed and Junior's parents, usually in response to everyone's distress, either slap or pull his hand away from his genitals. How does an infant understand this reaction? Once again, he is being taught that certain parts of his body are shameful or dirty. Parents must avoid such reactions. They need to be aware that infants live in a God-given world of sensual delight. Marriage and family counselor, Mary Ann Mayo says:

> The world of the normal infant includes orgasm, sometimes as a newborn, but always within the first year of life. Physically or emotionally deprived infants may rock, bang their heads, and excessively suck their thumbs, but they won't masturbate. It is the healthy child who involves himself or herself in genital play. The sad, emotionally, or physically deprived child does not bother.[2]

Allowing infants the freedom to explore their genitals should not be frightening to parents. It is simply one part of their learning experience. It will not become their major fascination. After awhile the baby's interest will center elsewhere. But your comfortable attitude regarding your child's genitals will have a calming effect and help him learn to accept his whole body.

Another area of physical importance in an infant's sex education is correctly naming the body parts. This is closely associated with parental acceptance of self-discovery. When allowing your child to explore the genital area just like other parts of the body, you should correctly name all the body parts. This will help you become comfortable using the proper names, and it will communicate acceptance of the whole body since all parts have been named and treated in the same way.

Another area of importance involves toilet training. Be patient and unhurried with regard to your infant's toilet training. If toilet training is attempted before an infant has the ability to voluntarily control the muscles involved in these functions, he will not be able to respond. Most child development experts agree that such control is rarely possible before the age of two or three years. Of course, you will discover that all of your relatives and friends had their babies completely toilet trained by age six months, and they do not mind constantly reminding you of that fact! Many years ago, with our first child, my wife was determined not to allow others to influence her decision to wait until our daughter was truly ready for toilet training. She waited until Stephanie was about two and a half years old. This caused somewhat strained family relations as she was the first grandchild on either side of the family. All of our relatives thought we were going to cause great mental anguish to our daughter and that she would probably go off to kindergarten in a diaper. But my wife stuck to her guns and did not begin until about 30 months.

Now you must understand, my wife is a very well-read and extremely creative person, and she does not do many things in the conventional manner. Toilet training was no exception—she began training Stephanie by placing the potty-chair in front of the television during children's shows such as "Sesame Street." Well, it only took a few days to completely toilet train our daughter. Everything was great until we had a house full of relatives one day and Stephanie got the urge. You guessed it! She ran into the bathroom, grabbed her potty-chair, set it down in front of the television and proceeded to do her business. She emptied the room in a hurry, and we had some explaining to do. But by waiting until she was ready, my wife had concluded an often very traumatic event in less than a week.

Have you ever seen a diaper-clad child in kindergarten? Probably not. But you have known many children who still wet their beds or wet their clothes in school. They are probably the ones who, through punishment and threats, were toilet trained by six months of age. Take your time in the toilet training of your child. By doing so you can avoid several potential emotional problems.

Hold, cuddle and physically touch your infant often. Babies show the most contentment when they are being held, rocked or in some way snuggled closely. Some babies appear to need more caressing than others, but all infants respond positively to relaxed, repeated caressing. When our son was about a year old he went through a stage where he very intensely needed to be held. He would not allow his mother or me to put him down for even an instant. Well, after a few days this grew rather old. Besides the physical weariness, we felt that by holding him constantly we were going to spoil him. So we put him down. After all, we had read Dr. Spock and we knew he, as well as other experts, said that a child would only cry for about ten minutes before going to sleep or finding some other interest. Our son had not read Dr. Spock! He cried for two solid hours and then began vomiting. This went on for two days! By this time Linda was at the end of her rope. In desperation she called a friend, a slightly older woman with older children.

After listening to the problem, this wise pastor's wife responded by asking Linda a question: "If your son had any other need what would you do?"

Linda said, "I would attempt to meet it."

The discerning lady then said, "Well he has a need to be near you right now, so why not meet that need?"

She then lent Linda a papoose-like backpack. For about a week Linda carried our son everywhere she went, and after that he was OK. Now, I'm not a doctor or a psychologist, and I do not presume to know all of the psychological factors at work in this situation, but I know at least one thing—during that particular time in his young life, our son needed a tremendous amount of physical intimacy. And I'm not sure he was much different from other infants.

Whatever we do that communicates a sense of warmth

and love to our babies, teaches them security and the enjoyment of physical intimacy. And security, warmth and love will help lay a foundation of self-confidence in our children, a vital element in the development of healthy sexual attitudes.

Allow your infants and toddlers to enjoy and learn about their bodies and the closeness of others. One way to accomplish this is by joining a swimming class for infants and parents. In this atmosphere children learn familiarity with their own bodies and the bodies of others. One of the best ways to help them achieve this bodily knowledge about themselves and others is to permit your young sons and daughters to bathe together. By bathing together children are not only learning about their own bodies but are also experiencing a natural lesson in the physical differences between males and females. In a nonthreatening, playful way children notice that their bodies are different. This could be one of those opportunities for teaching we talked about earlier. Parents can casually use such moments to begin teaching young children that God made people different, and that these differences have reasons. Around the age of five or so your children may begin requesting that they be permitted to bathe alone—it is time for some privacy. But for younger children, bathing together can produce perfect teaching opportunities.

In our discussion on important areas concerning our infants' sex education, we have up to this point stressed the "shoulds." Let's look at one "should not." Parents should not allow infants or toddlers to sleep in their room or bed with them. This not only restrains the parents' lovemaking, but it quite possibly causes the young child to become upset because of his lack of knowledge or understanding regarding his parents' behavior during lovemaking.

Sex Education for Preschoolers (Ages 2-5)

Physically speaking, the preschool years are years to continue building the concepts begun during the first year of your infant's life. It is important to continue using proper names for body parts, and to speak about human sexuality. The title of this book, of course, is a way to get you into the material, not a recommendation on how to talk to your kids.

In the area of toilet training and personal hygiene be sure to explain the reason for washing hands after using the potty. Help your toddlers to understand they are wiping properly and washing their hands to avoid carrying germs, not because that part of their body is shameful. This differentiation needs to be made so that the child will not think of the sex organs as dirty.

It is imperative that parents begin at birth to help children formulate a positive, healthy self-esteem.

It is essential during this critical stage that you continue appropriately touching your children. No one, male or female, ever outgrows the need to be touched. Continue to hug, hold and kiss your toddlers.

Preschool children can learn many negative emotions—shame, guilt, anger or fear—from their parents, in the process of learning about sex. Conversely, positive attitudes are taught when parents have wholesome, healthy, godly attitudes and teach about sex in a consistent and responsible way. Such positive teaching creates a loving, trusting bond between parent and child, and contributes greatly to laying a strong foundation of self-esteem. This is a vitally important aspect of sex education, since self-esteem, or the lack of it, profoundly affects all areas of child and adolescent behavior. "Promiscuous and exploitative sexual behavior, premature parenthood and a range of self-damaging behavior, feed off poor self-esteem."[3]

It is therefore imperative that parents begin at birth to help children formulate a positive, healthy self-esteem. Much of this is accomplished by doing the things we have already talked about: holding, cuddling, stroking, developing close physical contact, using gentleness and sensitivity when toilet training, and reacting positively to innocent, normal childhood sexual curiosity about their bodies. Children should never be punished or scolded because of innocent childhood sexual self-discoveries. When this is allowed to happen a whole range of negative emotional responses can occur: anger, withdrawal, fear, guilt—all adversely influencing self-esteem. Because of guilt and fear a child may learn to be dissatisfied with his body and become so disappointed that even as an adult sexual pleasure is impossible. Early childhood problems in this area leave scars, and while they can be healed, they are much more easily prevented.

Mentally and intellectually, the young child's belief system mirrors that of his parents. Children tend to believe what their parents believe. What attitudes and beliefs concerning sexuality are you teaching your children? Dr. Grace Ketterman, in her wonderful book, *How to Teach Your Child About Sex,* says that by school-age there are five attitudes your child needs to understand if he is to be a sexually healthy person.[4]

Attitude 1: *He needs to know that he is a beautiful child and that his imperfections only add to his uniqueness as a masterpiece created by God and nurtured by you.*

Repeatedly emphasize your unconditional love and your total and complete acceptance of your child. In this way your child begins to accept himself.

Attitude 2: *He needs to understand that every other person is also intended to be beautiful and unique and, therefore, to be respected as he respects himself.*

The second part of our Lord's great commandment was to "love your neighbor as you love yourself." Once again children will probably do no better or no worse in loving and appreciating others than their parents do. If we continually condemn, criticize and put others down, then our children will grow up with much the same attitude toward others. If we want our children to be understanding and compassionate toward others, then we must be their model.

Attitude 3: *He needs to know some of the physical differences between boys and girls and some facts about how babies are conceived and born.*

This can be accomplished, as we have already seen, by answering in a straightforward way the questions that naturally arise when swimming and bathing with members of the opposite sex. Obviously, the facts concerning conception that children need at this age are simple and basic. But this is the age to begin providing this knowledge.

Attitude 4: *He needs to have learned to respect the needs and feelings of others and to understand and resolve some of his own needs with the help of others.*

Once again parents are the key. When you show respect, not only for the needs and feelings of your children, but also for the needs and feeling of others, your children will observe and copy your behavior.

Attitude 5: *He needs to know how to accept children of either sex as friends, and how to interact with them socially in a way that is comfortable for both.*

The term friends here refers to playmates, and not boyfriend/girlfriend type relationships. Looking back over seventeen years in youth ministry one of the most disturbing trends I have observed is the growing tendency on the part of society to thrust young children into boy/girl relationships. Even some well-meaning parents try to push their children into such relationships at much too young an age. For the past ten years I have directed a summer church camp for children ranging in age from grades three to nine. One night during the week we have an old-fashioned campfire. It used to be that only the older kids, grades six through nine, worried about taking a person of the opposite sex to our campfire. However, during the last two years I have observed even the third graders starting to get anxious if they do not have someone to take to the campfire. I do my best to discourage this practice. There will be enough time for boy/girl relationships in the years ahead when their maturity level is high enough to handle such relationships. Please let your small children be children and learn to cultivate simple friend-ships. Dr. Ketterman also feels very strongly about this sub-ject. She says:

> It has come to be considered cute to tease very young children about having "boyfriends" and "girlfriends." It always surprises me that five- and six-year-olds seem to understand this as having sexual implications. They will bristle in anger, or they may laugh with those who tease, but they get the message that maybe they are supposed to start such relationships early. Childhood is very short at best, and it is sad to see it abbreviated even more by such teasing, with its implications. For many reasons, I urge you to avoid such teas-ing and caution your family or relatives to respect this policy.[5]

The phone rang late one afternoon. The young mother on the other end of the line was very distressed. She was almost in tears and desperately wanted some advice. She had just caught her daughter in the closet with their friend's son, and they were playing "doctor." That is to say they were satisfy-ing their natural curiosity concerning the bodies of the oppo-site sex. Now these children were only four and five, respec-tively, but this mother was convinced that they were both perverted and headed for a life of criminal sexual offenses. Her reaction was rather typical. Most parents are not pre-pared to handle this situation well and almost instinctively react very negatively. I very calmly tried to convince the mother that these children were quite normal, and that her reaction to this situation was the most critical issue at the moment. Fortunately, she had called me before responding to her child or her friend's child. I say, fortunately, because her first reaction, as she explained, was to punish her child severely, take her friend's child home and demand that he be punished also. In addition, she planned to break off all con-tact with her close friend.

I managed to soothe her fears by explaining that all children do some innocent experimenting at about this age, and that as long as she did not overreact it would cause no long-term damage to either child. I suggested that the best solution would be to take the children aside for a little chat. During this chat she should explain to them that their curiosity was normal, but perhaps a better way to find out about the body of the opposite sex would be for their parents to share this information with them, perhaps from a good book. I also cautioned the mother to discuss the subject calmly with the little boy's parents, taking care to explain what she had told both children. I assured her that most children outgrow such behavior after a short while, and that after the conclusion of this matter she would have successfully handled one of the biggest social aspects of her preschooler's sex education. I did not, however, have the heart to tell her that it gets worse in junior high!

Your preschooler also needs to learn about the spiritual aspect of sexuality. As Christian parents, we have the opportunity to teach our children about their sexuality in a biblical framework. The main lesson preschool children need to learn is that God created them, loves them, and cares deeply about them. They also need to know that they are a gift from God and are therefore very special. An excellent Scripture for children this age is Psalm 139:13-16. This very beautiful portion of God's Word tells children that they were created and formed in their mother's womb. Using this verse has two very important effects—it helps parents lay a basis for self-esteem that can be built upon for years to come, and it serves as a perfect introduction to the explanation of pregnancy.

Where Did I Come From?

Often before age five a child will ask the question—"Where did I come from?" Grasp the opportunity when it comes and tell your preschooler the wonderful story of the creation of life. Of course, the facts should be very elementary and commensurate with a small child's vocabulary and emotional level. You might say something like this:

> God loves children very much and He wants them born into a family with a mommy and a daddy. A baby needs a family to love him, talk to him, change his diaper and feed him. Little babies are totally helpless and the family is God's way of giving a baby a happy place to grow up and be loved.
>
> Inside a mother is a special place where babies grow. This place is like a tiny room and is called the womb or uterus. The baby starts growing in this special place when a tiny egg from inside the mother is joined with a tiny object from the father called the sperm. The egg and the sperm are so small you cannot see them without a magnifying glass. After they get together they grow in the womb. After a few weeks the egg has grown into a small baby with tiny arms and legs. After about three months the baby has fingers and toes. The baby grows inside the mother's womb for about nine months and when the baby is ready to be born he weighs about six or seven pounds and is about 20 inches long. The mother's body tells her when it is time for the baby to be born by beginning to squeeze, like you would squeeze your fist. When this happens the mother goes to the hospital for the baby to be born. The mother is helped at the hospital by a doctor. The squeezing keeps on pushing the baby from the mother's womb into another special place called the vagina. The vagina leads to the opening between the mother's legs, which leads to the outside world. The opening slowly stretches to let the baby out. The mother has some pain during the baby's birth, but the doctor helps and gives

the mother some medicine to help her and make her feel better.

Be sure to tell this amazing story with joy and happiness. Your attitude is as important as the facts you teach. This simple, accurate description of conception and birth will adequately satisfy your preschooler's curiosity. There will probably not be a need to discuss intercourse at this point because preschoolers are rarely interested in such details. But they are very interested in "where they came from."

Typical Questions Asked by Preschoolers

It is difficult to anticipate with any accuracy exactly the questions preschoolers will ask. Some children ask the expected questions right on schedule. Others appear uninterested until much later. But if you are an askable parent sooner or later your preschool children will ask a variety of questions. There are several questions that are frequently asked by children under six years of age. Generally speaking, the questions usually fall into two categories. At this age children are most concerned with body structure and function, and all matters relating to babies. It is OK to be very specific. Do not be afraid that you are furnishing too much information, because if your children need the facts you will have provided them, and if the information is over their heads, they will simply ignore it until a later date.

Children this age will ask about breasts, penises, belly buttons (umbilici), body hair and vaginas. In general, your answers need to center around the differences between boys and girls, and why God designed them differently. Explain that God's plan was for boys and girls to be different so that they could grow up to have bodies of men and women and become fathers and mothers.[6]

Here are some questions and possible answers:

Q. A little girl points to a penis and asks, "What's that, and why don't I have one?"

A. "It's a penis and little boys have penises for urination, and little girls have vulvas for the urine to get out of the body. God made boys and girls differently."

Q. "Why do mommies have big breasts and daddies don't?"

A. "Mommies breasts are bigger because God made mommies so they can make milk for babies."

Q. "Why is my penis not as big as daddy's?"

A. "As your entire body grows bigger, your penis will grow some too."

Q. "What's a vagina?"

A. "It's a special place a baby goes through to get out of the mother's body at birth."

As you can see questions of this type can be endless. Hopefully, your children will ask these questions of you rather than of relatives or strangers. When our son was about four years old he approached his paternal grandfather and very matter-of-factly said: "Daddy Bill, do you have a penis or a vagina?" My dad paused only briefly and replied: "A penis." Paul then said, "I thought so," and walked away. Fortunately my father knew, and approved of, our open style with our children.

Preschoolers also ask many questions related to birth and babies, especially if the mother becomes pregnant during this inquisitive age.

Q. "Can boys have babies?"

A. "No, it takes a daddy and a mommy to make a baby, but babies grow in the mommy."

Q. "Does it hurt to have a baby?"

A. "There is some pain—but God made mommies' bodies special so that with a doctor's help it doesn't hurt too much."

Q. "Did you know that I would be a boy (girl) before I was born?"

A. "Doctors have a special way to tell, but we just wanted you."

Answering your preschooler's questions simply and truthfully will begin the sex education process in an excellent manner. It will also teach your young child that you are approachable and askable, thus laying the foundation for an open communicating relationship with the child. From the beginning we have emphasized sex education as an ongoing process, beginning at the birth of your child. When you start this education at birth, you eliminate the pressure of finding and setting aside a special time for this purpose later. And by then the "staged" effect of the entire process becomes rather perfunctory. Starting early also lays the proper groundwork for better, more mature discussions as your child grows older. Your honest and open attitude with your preschooler will communicate your love and concern for him, and it will greatly increase the likelihood that your child will look to you for sexual information.

For Further Thought

1. What are your earliest recollections concerning your own sex education? Were your parents open and askable?
2. Which body parts are you the most uncomfortable naming correctly? How can you eliminate this uncomfortable feeling?
3. What type of example do you provide concerning the recognition of the needs and feelings of others? What improvements can you make?
4. What are some specific ways you can avoid having your young children pushed into boy/girl relationships before they are ready?
5. Have you ever caught one of your children playing "doctor" with another child? Were you pleased with your reaction? If it happened again how would you react differently?
6. Read Genesis 2:15-25. What explanations and observations regarding reproduction can be made using this passage?
7. What sexual questions can you anticipate your preschoolers asking? How would you respond?

Chapter 7

THE CAREFREE YEARS

(EARLY ELEMENTARY YEARS—AGES 6-9)

For children the early elementary school years (ages six through nine) are among the most carefree years of their lives. Physical growth has slowed considerably; parents provide most of their needs and wants; parents can be trusted, and puberty is an unknown enemy. The developmentally hectic preschool years seem far behind. During these early elementary years it even appears that sexual activity and interest is diminishing. This apparent disinterest in sex is caused partly because school considerably broadens their world. They now have many interests outside the home. Also, elementary age children are more easily embarrassed and therefore tend to conceal sexual activities and interests. Of course, appearances can be deceiving. Elementary children are still very concerned about their bodies and sexual matters. And many of the emotions, characteristics, habits and qualities learned during these seemingly dormant elementary years will have a significant impact on their adult sexuality. Parents should, therefore, remain active and aware as they look for opportunities to extend their children's sex education.

During this developmental stage children are much more comfortable with general rather than specific information. They are now able to express their feelings in words and can understand that a person does not act on every feeling. This new understanding reinforces competence and has a long-term effect on their sexual functioning. At this age children want honest, accurate answers to their questions and do not appreciate lectures. During this period, furnish accurate, dependable information in the context of open discussions. You should also express your opinions, communicate your values and be receptive to the personal needs of your child. Such an atmosphere will promote healthy sexual growth.[1]

Sexual Play (playing doctor) Is Winding Down

At the beginning of the elementary years, there may still be some mild sex play, such as "showing out" in school, but this type of behavior is in the process of easing off. And by age seven or eight it has slowed almost to a stop. As they outgrow "playing doctor," their curiosity about male/female body structure often manifests itself in their looking at nude or semi-nude magazine or catalog pictures. If this happens, do not overreact, but use the incident as an opportunity to teach self-respect as well as respect for others. These feelings and behavior are a normal part of growing up sexually.

Dirty Words and Smutty Jokes Are Winding Up

Just in case you were feeling relieved about sexual play decreasing, I need to inform you that dirty words, smutty jokes and writing sex phrases are your next concern. This kind of behavior usually begins about age six and starts with laughing or name-calling about bodily elimination. By age seven or eight, however, such behavior has increased and usually includes dirty or off-color jokes, writing sex words, calling other children sexual names (dick, prick, etc.), and attempting to peek at

girls. As children grow a little older this behavior escalates into
swearing, using sex words and phrases.[2] How are we to react to
such behavior? Should we grab the first bar of soap we see and
begin washing out our child's mouth? It depends on what has
been said and to whom.

Children should be taught that behavior such as name-calling, telling dirty jokes and publicly writing nasty words can
cause hurt feelings and embarrassing situations. They should
learn that above all, the feelings of others are always to be considered. They should also know that using shameful slang
terms for very beautiful God-given activities is not right. But be
careful not to overreact. Children at this age often use words
without knowing their full meanings. In addition, the words
may mean something different to your children than to you.

For example, when I was about twelve years old it was the
custom of my group of friends to refer to other boys as
"queers." One day I made the mistake of calling a boy a queer
in the presence of my dad! He was not pleased, and asked how
I knew that this boy was a homosexual? I was horrified. I barely knew what a homosexual was, and it was not my intention
to accuse this boy of anything like that. To my group of
friends, queer simply meant odd or weird. When I explained
to my dad, he understood, but he told me that not everyone
would see it that way. He suggested that if my friends and I
were going to use such terms, we do so in private, in order not
to hurt anyone's feelings. Most importantly, he did not overreact and have me shot.

I have tried to use the same approach with my son. I have
explained to him that I know he will use certain words and
terms while he is with his male friends, and that I will not
overreact as long as he respects the feelings of others and
avoids crude references to wholesome activities. I have also
explained to him that ladies are not pleased at even the hint of
crudity. Please do not misunderstand me. I am not suggesting
that you should condone filthy, dirty language. I am merely
suggesting that parents not overreact and that they gather all
facts before harshly punishing their children. Calm, rational,

controlled behavior speaks loudly to our children and keeps the door of communication open, and you can always increase discipline if the situation warrants.

Male/Female Body Structure

During these early elementary years boys and girls begin to be more aware of and interested in male/female body structure. And they maintain their interest in the bodies of the opposite sex even though they approach their physical natures differently.

The boys are very competitive and macho, and flex their scrawny muscles at each other. This competitive nature can

---

Even though elementary age boys and girls will never admit it, they maintain a high degree of interest in the body structure of the opposite sex.

---

lead to frequent fights and disagreements. As most mothers are no doubt aware, boys this age care little about appearance and see no need for daily showers or matching clothes. Boys of this age like any activity if it has two essential ingredients—it must be physical and it must be competitive.

Girls in this age group are vastly different from boys. They are very concerned with personal hygiene and matching outfits, including socks and hair ribbons. They compare hair, clothes, shoes and friends. They tend not to be as competitive as boys. (Whether the difference is cultural or biological is not known.)

Even though elementary age boys and girls will never admit it, they maintain a high degree of interest in the body structure of the opposite sex. Their rising self-consciousness, which begins shortly after entering school, prohibits "playing doctor." And they begin to become sensitive about exposing their bodies. As they move through the early elementary years their self-consciousness increases and may even develop to the extent that they do not want to be seen by the parent of the opposite sex. They are also highly susceptible to embarrassment concerning their bodies. This self-consciousness and embarrassment, coupled with their high interest in the bodies of the opposite sex, partly explains the peeking at each other and the looking at magazines. They are still very curious and want to see opposite sex bodies; they just do not want their own bodies seen.

Be aware of this increasing sensitivity and self-consciousness. Opposite sex parents should respect the privacy of their newly shy child. Also understand that although these children do not want to expose their own bodies, they may have no objection to everyone else in the family parading around partially clad. So if your family custom involves some nudity, do not change. I believe a certain amount of appropriate nudity is healthy. It teaches children that our bodies are not shameful or dirty.

Sex Roles and Identity

Just as this early elementary period is characterized by an increased awareness of male/female body structure, this period of development is also characterized by a dramatic increase in male/female role definition. Both sexes are becoming more conscious of what boys and girls are supposed to be and do. Therefore, it is extremely important for them to have sex roles defined and described. It is by learning what males and females are and do that a child begins to develop his own personal sexual identity. By sexual identity I mean the inner feelings by which a person can say "I feel like a male, or a female."[3] Sexual identity is very important as it defines sexual personhood for an individual.

During this early grade school period, children's awareness of what boys and girls are and do increases because of their exposure to television, radio, movies, printed media material, and by their observation of friends and family. Parents, however, should not depend on any of these, or other sources, to teach or define sex roles for their children. You need only watch television for a brief period to realize that our world does not hold godly values and teachings in very high esteem.

It is important that parents be the dominant provider of sex role information. Parents also need to understand that children do not learn sex role information by means of a short talk or lecture on the subject, but they learn these lessons, as they learn many others, by watching, observing and emulating their parents. Since children this age identify most strongly with the parent of the same sex, it is extremely important for same sex parents to be their children's role models and spend time with them. By observing same sex parents, children learn how this parent walks, talks, dresses, and even thinks. "It is vitally important for boys to identify with males and for girls

> Parents should attempt to break down sex role stereotypes; extreme stereotyping can lead to sexism and dehumanizing treatment of individuals.

to identify with females. Without such identification, children may later suffer sexual maladjustments."[4]

Parents should also attempt to break down sex role stereotypes, such as: "little boys don't play with dolls"; "boys don't cry, they're tough"; "girls do not participate in sports, it isn't ladylike"; "act like a man and be tough." Extreme stereotyping can lead to sexism and dehumanizing treatment of individuals. Unfortunately, much family violence is often a by-product of a family system that overemphasizes the traditional role of the authoritarian male and the submissive female. And, yes, I am aware of what God's word says in Ephesians 5: 22 and 25.

In verse 22 wives are told to "submit to your husbands" and in verse 25 husbands are told to "love your wives, just as Christ loved the church." The key words in these verses are "submit" and "love." A careful study of these words in the original language shows them to have almost the same meaning. Both the husband and wife are to submit to and love one another. These verses have been used too many years by abusive men attempting to justify their aggressive and dictatorial behavior. When men learn to love their wives "as Christ loved the church" the question of who is in charge will not seem so important.

One way parents can break down stereotyping is by having all family members participate in household chores. When women work outside the home, as many do, they are contributing in a financial way (traditionally a male role), and should not be required to do all the housework and cooking (traditionally a female role). In our home, for example, my schoolteacher wife is not responsible for all the household duties. Our children clean their rooms—at least twice a year—and I am responsible for cleaning the remainder of the house. Cooking chores are shared by my wife, my daughter and me. My wife also does the laundry and supervises homework. We are attempting to teach our children that everyone should contribute to our family and that stereotypical roles are not very important.

Please do not interpret any of the above discussion concerning sex role stereotyping as a suggestion that males and females have no differences and that we should adopt a unisex approach to life. I firmly believe God created male and female uniquely different, and that our children need to be taught the clear differences and distinctions between the sexes. I believe this can be done, however, in a nonexploitive manner.

Before leaving the subject of sex roles and the definition of these roles, a word concerning single parents is needed. It can be extremely frightening to rear children alone, especially opposite sex children. Mothers, who constitute the majority of single parents, are very concerned about meeting the needs of their sons. If you are a single parent and the absent spouse cannot or will not fulfill your child's role model needs, you must find adequate substitute role models. Young children need good relationships with same sex persons in order to develop an understanding of themselves as total, sexual beings. Such role models can be found in Big Brother, Big Sister Clubs, Boy and Girl Scouts and Little League. Mothers of sons can also request assignments to classes taught by men in both public and Sunday School.[5]

Single mothers also worry about not understanding their sons' emerging sexuality. They feel extremely inadequate about even knowing what to expect in terms of the sexual development of their sons. Space does not permit an extensive review of the subject here. However, in her book titled *Mothers and Sons,* Jean Lush provides a comprehensive list of the characteristics of a boy's sexual development.[6] This book and *Single Mothers Raising Sons* by Bobbie Reed, are both excellent resources for single mothers.

Boys and Girls?

At about age seven or eight children seem to have an instinctive awareness of their need to identify with same sex persons, and girls and boys begin increasingly to play separately. Boys gravitate toward select groups of peers and girls usually associate with one or two special friends. At this age the verbal banter between boys and girls begins. It is not uncommon for either sex to say that they "hate" boys or girls. Outwardly they appear to have no interest in the opposite sex, however, inwardly they are very much interested in sex and sexual matters. This is evidenced by the fact that despite the harsh words, they have crushes on members of the opposite sex, and they will admit to having boyfriends and girlfriends. Sexual interest is also confirmed by their sexual discussions and teasing with their same sex peers. Boys especially, engage in sexual discussions with their same sex friends. Girls generally talk much less about sexual matters with their girlfriends. This partly explains why boys this age may appear to be more knowledgeable about sexual matters.

During this time of apparent separation of the sexes, parents need to avoid teasing about boyfriends and girlfriends. Children this age are very sensitive and easily embarrassed by such teasing because they really believe they are showing no interest in the opposite sex. So be respectful and understanding concerning their boy/girl behavior.

We have already discussed the importance of the same sex parent in defining sex roles. Now the opposite sex parent receives equal billing. Opposite sex parents play a major role in helping their children develop comfortable and healthy attitudes toward children of the opposite sex. Children learn these comfortable attitudes by observing how their parents relate to each other and by receiving love and acceptance from both parents. It then becomes easier for children to give and receive love and trust from members of the opposite sex.

Opposite sex parents need to be involved in the lives of their children. Fathers need to take daughters shopping and spend time with them just as they spend time with their sons. Some of my fondest memories of my daughter's growing up years involve our semiannual shopping trips to Dallas. I would take her and several of her friends to buy school clothes, and we would hit all the big malls and make a day of it. We started this practice when she was in elementary school and continued right on through her high school years. Spending time with opposite sex parents lays the proper foundation for your children's future relationships with the opposite sex and it creates fond memories for mom and dad as well.

Increased Awareness of Pregnancy

At this age children begin associating pregnant women with babies, and their curiosity regarding pregnancy and birth increases. They often ask if the family is planning any new babies. They understand the process of pregnancy, and they become very curious about the father's role.[7] This stage is characterized by many questions about the origin, growth and birth of babies. In later elementary years, the questions concern conception. During this inquisitive period you should thoroughly explain conception. Respond to questions and actively create opportunities to talk even if there are no questions. If a new baby is born into the family at this time, an excellent opportunity exists for teaching. If not, consider visiting relatives or friends that have recently had babies. Such visits should provide excellent opportunities to teach these curious young minds.

Self-esteem

Self-esteem is a much discussed concept these days. Once while teaching a parenting class to a group of parents of junior high students, I was asked by a father if I blamed poor self-esteem for all of life's problems. The man was attempting to be sarcastic, and my answer probably startled him a bit. I told him that during all of my study and research, low self-esteem was always listed among the characteristics or reasons given for any deviant behavior (chemical dependency, eating disorders, juvenile delinquency, sexual experimentation) in adolescents. I further informed him that during many years in youth ministry, my own personal experience corroborated these findings. I am not saying that every child with a poor self-image will choose one or any of these deviant behaviors, but when one looks at any list of probable causes for all adolescent behavioral problems, a poor self-image is on every list! By poor self-image I mean self-esteem that is unusually low. All adolescents suffer from a slightly poor self-image during the transitional years of puberty. I have already said a great deal about building positive and strong self-esteem in our children, and more will follow. However, because of the importance of self-esteem and due to the teachable nature of children in the early elementary years, it is appropriate that we discuss it now.

Children of early elementary age are hero worshipers. Boys know the names and last year's statistics of any local quarterback or point guard. And girls know all the details about favorite actors and actresses. As children grow older their focus can become a favorite teacher, coach or pastor. Such hero worship helps children begin to select desirable traits they wish to acquire. The self-ideal is then centered on the question, "Who or what do I want to become." After determining a self-ideal, most adolescents consider a self-concept, their perception of what they are really like.[8] What children think of themselves is crucially important and their relationships will depend upon healthy self-esteem. Children tend to view others as they view themselves. And most importantly, they view themselves exactly as they are viewed by their parents. Parents are the prime creators of self-esteem in children. We can create either positive or negative self-images in our children.

In *Depression Hits Every Family*, Dr. Grace Ketterman lists twelve rules for building self-esteem in children. I have seen no better or more comprehensive list:

1. Develop an inner sense of unconditional acceptance of your child.
2. Practice communicating acceptance by listening, touching and spending time with them.
3. Explore their talents and interests.
4. Assign responsibilities to them.
5. Accept their friends.
6. Respect their ideas.
7. Respect and love their other parent.
8. Practice positive training and discipline.
9. Consistently express your approval and pleasure.
10. Teach and demonstrate forgiveness.
11. Teach your child to revel in all beauty.
12. Realize that your child has a mission in life.[9]

Take seriously your role as the principal provider of your child's self-esteem, and love your child.

Sexual Abuse and Molestation

After spending almost three decades working with teenagers, I am pretty well shockproof! However, one trend I have been observing over the past few years is both shocking and disturbing. I am amazed and saddened by the increasing number of child abuse or molestation cases that I uncover while counseling and working with young people. Our attitude toward child abuse has traditionally been that these things happen only among deranged or deprived people. But abuse is occurring with alarming regularity across all walks of life. The American Psychological Association estimates that between 12 and 15 million American women have been the victims of incest. A random sample of 930 San Francisco women revealed that 28 percent had been sexually abused before age 14.[10] Our focus in this book is on how to talk to and help our children. Therefore we must give some consideration to preparing our children in the event that someone may try to molest or abuse them. Hopefully, we can prepare our children in such a manner that they will be able to prevent such abuse or, if necessary, successfully recover from such an occurrence.

First, it is important to know that children are most often abused by a relative or friend that is known to them. Usually both the parent and the child have a certain amount of trust for the person. Of course, there are cases of total strangers abducting and abusing children, but these cases represent only about 25 percent of the offenses.

Secondly, if child molestation does occur, parents should not blame or accuse the child in any way. The child has experienced enough pain and trauma. Not only is it damaging to the child to be accused or blamed, it is totally absurd because children (especially small children) do not have enough understanding of sexual matters to have contributed in any way to the situation. Parents should remain calm and cool and immediately seek professional help.

In order to prepare your children (boys and girls need equal preparation) for any eventuality, the following items should be covered:

1. Warn your children specifically about molestation, describing some detail. The object is not to scare them, but to help them see the seriousness of the situation.
2. Help them develop a plan. This plan should include details of escape, emergency phone numbers and specific things to say.
3. Tell them that at their age no one has a right to touch their genitals, and they have every right to say no, and get away.
4. Explain to them that, while not everyone is evil, some people are bad. Further explain that they do not have to talk to people of that type.
5. Tell them if all else fails, scream for help!

6. Tell them that they can and should tell you everything, even if they were threatened and they promised not to tell!

Child abuse hotlines and abuse centers exist in every state. A major nationwide provider of such services is Parents Anonymous (PA) 1 800 421-0353, in California 1 800 352-0386.

Remember, that how well a child adapts after a crisis such as sexual abuse depends on how well *you* respond to the situation!

Typical Questions Asked by Early Elementary Children
In the early elementary school grades children's questions about reproduction continue to focus on the baby's origin, growth inside the mother, and entrance into the world. At this age children are very interested in the differences between males and females. Obviously the depth of this interest is greater than during the preschool years. Here are some of the most frequently asked questions concerning male/female differences, and the origin and growth of babies.
Questions:

Q. Do all women have babies?

A. No, only women who have had sexual intercourse.

Q. Can boys and girls, like Billy and I make a baby, and can I have a baby?

A. Such a question is common during the early elementary years and usually indicates an incomplete understanding of the reproductive process. You should explain that girls can only start having babies after they start to menstruate. Explain menstruation in simple terms if necessary. Also explain that people usually wait until they are married and old enough to care for a baby before they have one.

Q. How does a baby get out of mommy's stomach?

A. First of all, the baby is not in mommy's stomach. It stays in a special place called the uterus. When the baby is ready to be born it comes out through the vagina. The vagina stretches so the baby can come out. Explain that sometimes there are special problems and the doctor takes the baby out by a special operation. A brief, simple, explanation of a cesarean section, is in order.[11]

Q. How does a baby get started? Or how does the daddy put his sperm into the mother?

A. Of course, this is the dreaded "big" question. It will usually not be asked until about eight or nine. By this time children are ready for an honest, factual answer. Actually, straightforward honesty in answering this question, while embarrassing to the parent, is preferable to some of the wild imaginative stories children create in their minds. Your children will appreciate the honesty, and they will be properly informed during the critical years of puberty. Answer like this:

God designed the bodies of mothers and fathers to fit together in a special way. The Bible calls this "one flesh" because they join together. The father joins with the mother by placing his penis inside the mother's body in the vagina. This is called making love, or intercourse. The sperm from the father's body joins with an egg from the mother's body and a baby is started.

Q. Is intercourse or sex a sin?

A. This, or a similar question could easily follow the above question. Simply say: God created sex and He made men and women want to have intercourse so they could have children, and have fun together. God's Word, the Bible, tells us that sex is supposed to be for married people. When unmarried people have sex, then it is a sin.

Q. Do you and daddy have sex?

A. Probably a follow-up to the two previous questions. Answer: "Yes."

Q. Do boys have periods?

A. No, only girls. Boys go through other physical changes to prepare to be fathers.

It would be impossible to discuss all the questions children this age could ask. Their little minds can think of millions of questions, all seemingly designed to make parents squirm. But when children have been openly, honestly and lovingly told about sexual matters since birth, they will accept this new information in a natural way. It will be seen by them as natural and loving, not dirty and shameful. Remember—your attitude is the key.

For Further Thought

1. Anticipate your responses to your eight year old when he says, "Boy, that's lousy, it really sucks!"
2. Think about your family's practices concerning nudity. Are they appropriate? What are these practices communicating to your children?
3. What specific activities are done with your same sex children alone?
4. What sexual stereotypes bug you? Why?
5. What do you teach your children regarding the roles of males and females?
6. Father, what activities do you enjoy with your daughter? How often are these done? (Mother—son).
7. What specific things could you do to strengthen your child's self-esteem? What possible self-esteem needs of your children do you find hardest to meet?
8. Have you discussed sexual molestation with your children? Devise a plan for such a talk.
9. Does your early elementary (ages 6-9) age child understand intercourse? Think of opportunities to provide teaching on the subject.

Chapter 8

YOU'RE PREPARING ME FOR WHAT?
(PRETEEN YEARS—AGES 10-12)

To begin with, it sounds weird or strange. Say it out loud: puberty. See! It sounds like something you would step in and then say, "Oh, no, now I've got puberty all over my shoes." Well, it not only sounds weird, most of the time it is!

Once a year I am invited to a local Christian school to show a film about puberty and sexuality, and then to answer questions from several classes of fifth grade boys. This enlightening event follows several weeks study of James Dobson's *Preparing for Adolescence*. After these young men are taught this course about puberty by their female teachers, they are rewarded by watching a film and having their questions answered by me! I don't think I'm invited to this film screening and hot seat session because I'm an expert—the school just figures I'm the only one dumb enough to answer sex questions from fifth grade boys for an hour.

Several years ago, a smallish-looking fifth grader, after com-

pleting the course and watching the film, had apparently
heard enough about puberty. He raised his hand in response to
my invitation for questions, and said, "Mr. Talley, this puferty
(*that's right, puferty*) thing has got me kinda scared, isn't there
something we could take?" Well, what could I say? "Puferty," I
mean puberty, is pretty scary. I know many parents who would
gladly pay huge sums of money for "something to take" when
it comes time for their children to enter the mysterious world
of puberty. Puberty, next to birth itself, is the most drastic
change we experience in life, but unlike birth, we are actually
aware of the exciting transition through which we pass.[1]

Puberty can be a fearful experience even when the young
people are aware of what is happening. But children between
the ages of ten and twelve typically do not have any conception of the tremendous changes that will shortly occur in their
minds and bodies. Puberty is frightening at best, but if a child
is totally unprepared for the traumatic events that accompany
this developmental stage, major physical and emotional problems may be expected. Thus, your primary role during these
preteen years (ages 10-12) is to prepare your child thoroughly
and adequately for puberty.

At this point you may be thinking that 10-, 11- and 12-year-
olds are too young for a discussion of puberty, and that there
will be plenty of time as they grow older for such discussions.
But because of better nutrition, and for several other reasons,
young people are maturing physically earlier and earlier. For
example, in the 1870s the average girl first menstruated when
she was 16 or 17. In the 1980s she is more likely to menstruate
at 12 or 13. At this time in the United States, the average age
for the onset of menstruation is 12.9 years. In 1870 the average
age of puberty was 16.5. Today the average age of puberty is
about 12.5.[2]

Some children, especially girls, begin the first physical signs
of puberty as early as nine. In fact, 95 percent of all girls show
at least one sign of puberty between the age of nine and thirteen and a half. So it is important to begin preparing children
for the changes of puberty much earlier than in years past. Of

course, no two children will begin puberty at precisely the same age, so you need to be watchful and sensitively aware of your own child's particular physical timetable.

Before we proceed further, a definition of puberty is in order. Puberty may be defined as the period or age when one is capable of sexual reproduction. A person's body experiences primary changes which are internal and involve the reproductive organs, and secondary, or external, changes which involve outward physical appearances. The only difference between prepubescent children is that girls may be slightly taller than boys. Before puberty, however, boys and girls tend to look much alike physically. But this similarity is about to be radically altered.

Help, Something Is Happening to My Body!

During puberty children's bodies go through tremendous changes. These changes often occur very rapidly, and children do not have time to adjust to one change before they are attacked by another. Physically speaking, most boys and girls mature into men and women before they leave junior high school. And the major physical changes that occur during puberty have a tremendous impact on the child's emotions.

Female puberty

For girls the physical changes that frequently cause the most concern or misunderstanding are: noticeable changes in height, weight and hips; appearance and development of breasts; menstruation and body shape.

For girls a sure sign of approaching puberty is the noticeable acceleration in both height and weight gain and a widening of the hips. Growth in height usually begins the process, and as early as nine or ten years old, girls usually begin to outgrow boys. Girls' growth spurts usually start about two years before those of boys. On the average, growth in height for girls begins at age ten and a half and is usually over by age 14. As this growth spurt begins, the girl usually experience a widening of the hips and an increase in body fat. This results in her becoming rounder and softer, and she may become very concerned about her shape and figure. Other physical changes include: growth of pubic hair, a slight deepening of the voice and increased activity in the sweat glands.

The appearance of breasts is usually the first sign that puberty is in high gear. Breast development usually begins between the ages of 8 and 13 and is normally over between the ages of 15 and 18. It is unfortunate that our society is pre-occupied with breasts and equates sexual desirability, and even femininity, with large breasts. Because of this fetish, many girls with small breasts suffer real mental anguish because they believe they compare unfavorably with other girls and thus boys will not like them. This extraordinary sensitivity to breast development is one of the most traumatic worries of puberty for girls.

Another problem associated with breast development occurs when girls' breasts develop early. When young girls develop large breasts, they may become the target of comments and stares from older boys and men, as well as teasing and harassment from other girls. Such attention from older boys can cause some major problems. It can cause fear and trauma, or it can encourage early sexual experimentation and promiscuity. Remember that physical maturity does not signal emotional maturity and breast size has no relation to a young girl's ability to relate maturely to older boys. If your daughter's physical time clock races ahead of her emotional/judgmental/cognitive time clock, do not hesitate to slow the clock. Insist that your daughter be treated in a manner appropriate to her age, regardless of her physical endowments. When we talk about dating, we will discuss the effect of a girl's early physical development on older boys. However, for now let me say that at this age such relationships with older boys should not be allowed.

Teenagers need to be reassured and helped to accept themselves just as they are. Use this time to reinforce the positive self-esteem they have been building since birth, not to validate the world's warped value system.

The most widely known and important aspect of puberty for girls is the onset of menstruation. This event usually occurs about two years after breast development and after the peak period of growth in height. As mentioned earlier, the average age for beginning menstruation is 12.9 years, but it can occur any time between ages nine and 18 years. Every preteen girl needs to understand and be prepared for this very special event before it begins. Mothers need to watch their daughter for signs of physical change such as: growth of pubic hair, rapid height gain and breast development. These events usually precede menstruation by at least one year, and sometimes as much as three years.

In addition to observing your daughter's physical changes, it is important to have at least introduced the topic of birth during the early elementary age years. Associating menstruation with matters related to babies and birth is natural, and by routinely discussing the topic at this time, a mother will be preventing complete surprise on her daughter's part in the event of an early beginning of menstruation. In any case, as soon as you suspect that your daughter is approaching puberty, discuss menstruation with her and tell her exactly what to expect. Explain the process of menstruation thoroughly and provide complete, accurate information regarding menstrual care and personal hygiene. With today's modern advances producing thinner pads and smaller tampons, menstruation does not cause the discomfort of years past. And even the smallest girl should be able to wear tampons.

Menstrual cycles for young adolescent girls can vary and be irregular at times, and the length of periods and amount of flow varies with each individual. Young girls' periods can also be affected by stress, diet, illness and exercise. Of course, persistent problems with a girl's menstruation process should be quickly brought to the attention of a doctor. A physician should be consulted if: the hymen is completely closed preventing the use of tampons; the menstrual cycle is still irregular two years after the first period; there is excessive bleeding with periods (soaking pads), there is bleeding between periods;

the girl experiences excessive cramping and a tendency to faint during periods.[3]

Girls should also be prepared for the physical pain that can precede and continue through the period. This pain is usually the result of fluid retention by the body. The degree and length of pain varies with each girl. The swelling usually occurs about a week prior to the menstrual period, and will generally produce a feeling of physical heaviness and emotional tension. At the age of 10 to 12 the physical pain and discomfort of menstruation should not be overemphasized. However, young girls approaching puberty should be calmly counseled and advised concerning PMS (premenstrual syndrome) and the physical discomfort often associated with menstrual periods.

No matter how much preparation you have given your daughter, expect her still to be somewhat embarrassed during her first periods. At the start of menstruation a girl may worry that blood can soak through her clothing, or that the outline of her sanitary pad can be seen through her clothes. She may also fear a bad odor. All of these concerns are related primarily to the dreaded fear that somehow boys may know she is menstruating. Because they are concerned that boys may become aware of their condition, young girls may refuse to attend parties or other social activities. Mothers need to reassure their daughters that their periods are not so easily detectable. Girls should be encouraged to change pads and tampons frequently to eliminate any small possibility of staining. This should relieve their fears. Above all, a young girl experiencing menstrual periods for the first time needs calm reassurance that this strange, new, apparent inconvenience, is completely normal, healthy and clean. It's a sign from God that she is becoming a woman. Your positive attitude will provide comfort and support, and will help ensure your daughter's positive attitude toward this new change in her body.

It is the opinion of most experts that boys also need an understanding of the menstruation process. It is not inappropriate to discuss this process in mixed groups of males and females. But even if mixed group discussions seem inappropriate, boys need some teaching on this subject. Such teaching helps boys understand what is happening to young ladies and why. And it could help boys avoid embarrassing situations in future mixed company events. I think it is important that boys be taught to respect the privacy of this occurrence, and to be respectful and not ridicule or make fun of girls during their periods. I often hear teenage boys and girls openly discussing menstruation, and I am amazed at their crudity and flippant attitude. It is not uncommon for boys to blame every single instance of anger, frustration and stress on menstruation. They say things like "she's on the rag, you better avoid her", or "it's the wrong time of the month, you better watch out." Teenage girls even join the seemingly harmless banter regarding menstruation. It is my opinion that such an attitude, while it is not meant to be harmful or degrading, is in most cases inappropriate and should be avoided. Boys, especially at this age, should be learning how to treat ladies. And I constantly tell my teenage son, "All women are ladies, whether they know it or not, and they should be treated in a dignified, kind manner." Harmful put-downs and demeaning of female peers is not good preparation for being a thoughtful, loving, Christian husband.

Male puberty
For a boy the physical changes that cause the most worry and misunderstanding are: lack of growth in height and weight, body hair, the size of his penis, spontaneous erections and wet dreams.

A boy's first worry related to puberty is that he is not growing as fast as the girls his age. Height is extremely important to boys because they consider it a visible sign of manhood and a way of attracting girls. On the average, boys' growth in height lags behind that of girls by about two years. Their growth spurt usually begins about age 12 (although it can begin as early as ten and a half or as late as 17), is most rapid at age 14, and is usually concluded at age 16. For boys who grow tall rapidly, the problems of puberty are greatly diminished, but for the late developer, height can easily become the major concern of puberty. Boys who remain shorter than their peers during puberty are extremely self-conscious and need parental support and encouragement in order to bolster their sagging self-esteem.

One of the most revealing signs of approaching puberty for boys is the appearance of pubic hair. For boys, pubic hair corresponds in significance to breast development for girls. Boys who acquire pubic hair early are the envy of their peers, and often show off this new growth by parading around the locker room nude. Conversely, boys who are late growing pubic hair will rarely even undress in front of their friends. Parents need to be as sympathetic toward boys who are late to grow pubic hair as they are toward girls who develop breasts late. Late development in either case can be very traumatic for adolescents. With the development of pubic hair comes other body hair, especially under the arms and on the face. And by about 16 or 17 boys gradually need to begin shaving. Other physical changes that occur during puberty are: a deepening of the voice, increased activity of the sweat glands, growth and development of the muscle tissue, and acne.

A boy's testicles and penis begin growing at about age eleven and a half or some time between the ages of 10 and thirteen and a half. This growth continues for approximately three or four years. One of the greatest concerns for boys is the growth in the size of the penis. The penis grows rapidly about a year after the growth in the testicles has begun, and pubic hair has appeared. This growth continues until ages thirteen and a half to sixteen and a half. The average penis size is between four and six inches in a flaccid state. Because there is so much erroneous and mythical information about penis size, let me quote an authority on the subject:

> The size and the shape of the penis are not related to a man's physique, race, virility, or ability to give or to receive pleasure. Like any organ, penises differ

in size, but the differences tend to diminish in the
erect state. The penis neither atrophies with lack of
use nor enlarges through frequent use.[4]

Parents should furnish their adolescent boys with accurate
information of this kind because they have many fears and
worries concerning the size of the penis. Your awareness and
understanding can be most beneficial.

Some time between the ages of 13 and 16 a boy's testicles
can produce sperm. A boy's penis has been capable of erection
since birth, but as a child his erections were most likely in
response to rubbing or physical stimulation. Toward puberty
his penis is likely to become erect readily and frequently. This
may occur spontaneously or in response to sexually provoca-
tive sights, sounds, smells and fantasies. His erections are likely
to be accompanied by strong feelings of sexual desire.[5] These
physical changes and new sexual desires cause the dreaded
unwanted erections. And the unwelcome erections seem always to occur at the most inopportune times, the resulting
bulge in a boy's pants causing great embarrassment. Fathers
should prepare their sons for such occurrences by explaining
and warning them beforehand and providing warm, sensitive
support and understanding.

Another possibly traumatic occurrence for pubescent boys
is their first ejaculation. This usually happens during sleep and
is referred to as a nocturnal emission (wet dream). Prior to
puberty, even when experiencing sexual dreams or fantasies,
ejaculation was not possible. But following the physical
changes of puberty, ejaculation is now possible and sometimes
occurs during the sleeping hours. For the completely unprepared boy, much worry and guilt often accompanies his first
wet dream. In addition to not understanding what has happened, he may experience guilt, somehow believing his lustful
dreams are sinful. You should thoroughly prepare your prepubescent boy for this event, explaining that nocturnal emissions are the body's way of releasing sexual tensions and
preparing for sexual intercourse during marriage. Your son

should be told that this is all part of God's plan for his approaching manhood, and that he should not feel guilty.

Help Me! (What Parents Can Do)

Throughout our discussion on physical changes of puberty, we have alluded to the emotional concerns and worries of adolescents. It is very common for adolescents to compare themselves to their peers and to then be embarrassed and feel inferior. Girls compare their breasts and overall figures. Boys compare height, muscles and penises. The reason that these com-

---

You can build self-esteem by repeatedly explaining and modeling to your children that personal worth is determined by who they are inside...not beauty and/or athletic ability.

---

parisons are made is that physical appearances are very important because they dramatically affect the social life of the adolescent. Beginning at puberty or about junior high age, a very inflexible social system emerges. Unfortunately this system has only two groups—popular and unpopular. Popular boys are the early-developed athletic types. Popular girls are the pretty and full figured ones. To be short, fat, flat-chested, plain and nonathletic is to be permanently assigned to the unpopular group.[6] Is it any wonder that pubescent children attach so much importance to physical appearance? There are some things we can do to help our children overcome their fears and worries concerning their bodies, and prevent their self-images from plunging to new lows during this time of early puberty.

1. *Prepare them adequately.* The key issue is: no surprises! When I was about 16 my younger sister began menstruation. I was the oldest child and was baby-sitting my sister and two younger brothers. My sister was only about eleven and a half. Consequently, she had not been prepared for the event. There we were. She was not sure if she was bleeding to death, and even though I knew what was happening, I was not able to explain adequate-

ly or show her how to take care of herself. Make sure you eliminate the possibility for surprises by preparing your children for all that lies ahead of them. To eliminate their fears of being left out of the puberty process, be sure you explain to them that all people are different, and that physical development may be faster for some and slower for others. Assure them that their time is coming, and that they *will* experience puberty.

2. *Look for ways to build self-esteem.* You can build self-esteem, or at least keep it from diminishing, by repeatedly explaining and modeling to your children that personal worth is determined by who they are inside, and is not dependent upon beauty, social position, and genital or breast size. Continually seek ways to build self-esteem based on your child's inner strengths. Be on the lookout for ways to affirm your children by looking for ways in which they can excel. This is especially important for slow physical developers who may not be receiving affirmation based on beauty and/or athletic ability.

3. *Remember and relate your struggles.* Do you remember your own battle and struggles with puberty? Do you remember the embarrassment and the feelings of inferiority? Were you an early or late developer, and what struggles did you have with acne, unwanted erections or guilt over sexual feelings? Share these struggles with your children. They need to understand that even though you are now a confident, competent adult, you experienced the same struggles going through puberty as they are experiencing. By sharing your struggles with your children you are communicating three very needed messages: (1) You are telling your children that they are completely normal. Everyone experiences feelings of inferiority, embarrassment and guilt. (2) You are also communicating that you are aware of their concerns and that you are sensitive to their feelings and needs. (3) You are giving your children hope. You are saying to them "Yes, it's a struggle, but you can and will survive." They see that,

despite your struggles with puberty and all its accompanying problems, you developed into a mature, competent adult.

4. *Avoid embarrassing your children.* Pubescent children experience enough cruel jokes and put-downs from their peers that they certainly do not need any embarrassing remarks from their parents. Although they can usually survive being made fun of by their peers, the ridicule of a parent has a particularly stinging effect. Especially avoid embarrassing them in front of their peers. Advice, correction and embarrassing suggestions should be made in private.

5. *Respect their privacy.* As children enter the years of puberty, privacy becomes very important to them. They suddenly begin locking the bedroom and bathroom doors. Respect this new need for additional privacy and encourage other family members to be sensitive to these needs. Respecting children's privacy also conveys to them that you are being responsive to their feelings.

6. *Distinguish between temptation and sin.* We have already mentioned the potential for guilt in adolescent boys over unwanted erections, wet dreams and sexual thoughts. To keep your son's guilt from becoming unbearable, make a clear distinction between temptation and sin. When the Bible talks about lust, it is not talking about fleeting sexual thoughts. The word for lust is a very strong word meaning to "greatly desire." It does not mean just noticing that a person is sexually attractive and having momentary sexual thoughts. God created humans as sexual beings capable of sexual arousal. It is natural, therefore, that people will have sexual thoughts and become aroused. Sin occurs only if we dwell on the matter and intentionally think about it repeatedly. Be sure that your sons can distinguish between temptation and sin. Being able to make this distinction will eliminate a great amount of unrealistic guilt for our sons.

7. *Communicate unconditional love and forgiveness.* This has

been mentioned previously, but as parents we cannot be told too often to communicate unconditional love and practice forgiveness. When our children know that come what may they will always be loved, the burdens of puberty become bearable. What better way to enhance your child's self-esteem than to say, "I will love you no matter what, and please forgive me." Always remember, "love covers a multitude of sins."

Masturbation: Curse, Sin or Gift?

One of the most traumatic sexual problems of childhood is masturbation. The very mention of the word causes some people to cringe and become emotionally upset. This is due to the many fears, prejudices and myths surrounding this misunderstood and controversial subject. It is vitally important for parents to be knowledgeable on the subject of masturbation. Your knowledge should include an understanding of the psychological and emotional effects on children and teenagers. You should also be aware that the Christian community is divided on this subject. I am not attempting to provide an authoritative answer regarding this very controversial subject. Rather, I will furnish you with accurate information and the opinions of a wide range of Christian ministers, writers, psychologists and doctors.

First of all, let us properly define masturbation. It is easy to see why so many people have a very negative opinion of masturbation because the very word came from the Latin word that means "to pollute with the hand."[7] Masturbation is literally the act of stimulating one's own genitals by touching or caressing, usually to the point of orgasm or climax. During masturbation, sexual pleasure is experienced alone, without a partner. Boys usually masturbate by holding the penis in the hand and moving it up and down until the point of ejaculation. Girls in their early adolescent years typically do not have a strong need for genital sexual release but when girls do masturbate it involves rubbing the vulval area, especially the clitoris. A recent survey suggests that about 85 to 90 percent of teenage boys masturbate and that 50 to 60 percent of girls do the same. Boys start masturbating earlier than girls, with 50 percent engaging in the practice by age 13. Only 37 percent of teenage girls are masturbating at that age.[8]

In the not too distant past, masturbation was universally regarded as filthy, offensive and physically, psychologically and spiritually detrimental and damaging. Masturbation was said to cause insanity, deafness, blindness and acne. Boys were told "your penis will fall off," "hair will grow in the palms of your hands," "you will use all your semen," or "your face will become covered with zits." Girls were told that masturbation diminished their ability to bear children. In the 1920s and 1930s children were severely punished, and in some cases fitted with specially designed chastity belts to prevent masturbation. Obviously the practice of masturbation was frowned upon.

Today, however, we live in a much more liberated and enlightened age. It is now admitted and recognized that masturbation is not physically harmful. As far as psychological harm is concerned, many psychologists and sex educators believe that the only harm caused by masturbation is the massive guilt that many young people have because of this practice. Many suggest that masturbation is one way adolescents can safely and harmlessly relieve sexual tension. Others suggest that since our society typically encourages later marriages, long after the time of peak sexual intensity for males, masturbation is a natural consequence. Those taking this view believe that masturbation is a far better and more acceptable outlet for sexual release than acts of promiscuity and fornication. On the other side of the coin, there are those in the Christian community who strongly believe that masturbation is harmful and sinful. Those accepting this view believe that masturbation is harmful because: it originates in lust and fantasy, it becomes obsessive, it is self-pleasuring and selfish; and it causes homosexual tendencies.

These are some of today's prevailing views on masturbation. But as we have stressed before, parents must be very careful and selective about accepting or rejecting popularly held views on sexual matters. So what should we tell our children with regard to masturbation? And does the Bible address this subject?

As I said, Christian authors and ministers vary widely in their views on masturbation. There seems to be a continuum of opinion ranging from "masturbation is a sin in God's sight" to "masturbation is a gift of God." Let's examine the main viewpoints held by contemporary Christian writers and professionals.

Among some Christian writers, ministers, and professionals there is the view that masturbation is sin. It is viewed as lust and fantasy and is therefore sin. As proof they often refer to Genesis 38:6-10 and 1 Cor. 6:9. In Genesis, chapter 38, we find the story of Onan. Onan "spilled his semen on the ground." A careful reading of this passage, however, reveals that Onan's sin was not masturbation. He was simply practicing coitus interruptus. In other words, Onan withdrew before ejaculation. His sin was his refusal to provide children for his dead brother as commanded by Jewish law. In 1 Cor. 6:9. (KJV) it says "abusers of themselves with mankind." Some believe that self-abuse is masturbation. But a careful reading of this verse in either a modern language translation or an original language text reveals this phrase to be referring to homosexual behavior.[9] The Bible simply does not talk about it.

A second group of Christian professionals looks upon masturbation as wrong because it involves lust, fantasy and obsessive behavior, and it does not meet God's intentions for sex. These people believe that lustful thoughts are enough to condemn the practice of masturbation, and that it produces selfish and obsessive behavior. They argue that practiced excessively it can become idolatrous and, thus, sinful. Mary Ann Mayo in *Parent's Guide to Sex Education* raises doubts about this argument: "We all know people who don't function well or who have become idolatrous toward their jobs, money, position, their 'mission'. Do you really know anyone whose life centers around masturbation?"[10]

In a third category are those Christians who suggest that masturbation may be a way of releasing sexual tensions. They suggest that masturbation may be a God-given way to avoid premarital or extramarital sexual intercourse, as well as decrease lust and excessive sexual fantasies. One leading proponent of this view, Charles Shedd, speaks of masturbation as "the wise provision of a very wise creator. Something God gave us because he knew we'd need it."[11]

Many leading Christian psychologists, psychiatrists and counselors during the past ten years have reached similar conclusions regarding masturbation. They view it as a normal part of adolescence that, generally speaking, can safely relieve sexual pressures. They see masturbation as much preferable to premarital sex. These experts believe, however, that masturbation may become harmful or counterproductive when it becomes an obsessive or compulsive habit. They also feel that though masturbation is not a sin, the lustful thoughts that usually accompany the act may be sinful if these thoughts become compulsive. When obsessive behavior results from masturbation, either physically or mentally, there is also the issue of self-control.[12] These experts suggest a cautious approach when dealing with children and teenagers concerning masturbation. They suggest such an approach because of the strong feelings of guilt and anxiety that masturbation can produce in adolescents. Dr. James Dobson in *Preparing for Adolescence*, speaks to the adolescent from a Christian perspective. In my opinion parents should copy both the style and content of Dr. Dobson's message:

> The subject of masturbation is a very controversial one. Christian people have different opinions about how God views this act. Unfortunately, I can't speak directly for God on this subject, since His Holy Word, the Bible, is silent at this point. I will tell you what I believe, although I certainly do not want to contradict what your parents or your pastor believe. It is my opinion that masturbation

is not much of an issue with God. It's a normal part
of adolescence which involves no one else. It does
not cause disease, it does not produce babies and
Jesus did not mention it in the Bible. I'm not
telling you to masturbate, and I hope you won't
feel the need for it. But if you do, it is my opinion
that you should not struggle with guilt over it.[13]

In addition to cautiously and lovingly explaining masturbation to your adolescent, these experts suggest that you actively

---

> Adolescents need to find outlets—athletics,
> strenuous work and hobbies—for releasing
> emotional tensions caused by their sexual drives.

---

help your children keep masturbation from becoming obsessive and uncontrolled. This can be done by helping them
avoid sexually stimulating movies, television, books, magazines and music. Help your adolescents find other outlets—
athletics, strenuous work and hobbies—for releasing emotional
tensions caused by their sexual drives.[14] You should also
strongly discourage young boys from masturbating in groups.

In summary, leading experts view masturbation as a normal
part of an adolescent's development. They advise parents
against placing additional guilt on their children when dealing
with this issue. When abuses or excesses occur, parents should
respond with a wholesome, loving attitude that will relieve
guilt and promote healthy sexual attitudes.

Subjects that Should Be Discussed Prior to Puberty

In response to the question: "What should I talk about when I
discuss sex with my preteenager?" Dr. James Dobson gave the
following list of subjects:

1. The role of intercourse in marriage.
2. Male and female anatomy and physiology.
3. Pregnancy and the birth process.
4. Nocturnal emissions ("wet dreams").

5. Masturbation.
6. Guilt and sexual fantasy.
7. Menstruation.
8. Morality and responsibility in sex.
9. Venereal disease.
10. Secondary sex characteristics which will be brought about by glandular changes—pubic hair, general sexual development, increasing interest in sex, etc.[15]

Most of these subjects have been discussed in this book. The one exception is number nine on the list—venereal disease. Preteen children need to be introduced to the general topic of sexually transmitted diseases (STD). Specific, detailed information regarding venereal disease should be handled during early adolescence (ages 13-15).

Final Word

Puberty represents one of the most stressful times of life. Even at its best it produces physical and emotional trauma. When children have been thoroughly and adequately prepared for this stressful and traumatic stage of life, they will adjust and mature with a much healthier self-esteem. You need to lovingly provide your preteens with accurate information concerning all aspects of puberty. Of particular importance is your own acceptance of the confused feelings and emotions of adolescents during puberty. With accurate information and the loving acceptance of their parents, most children can successfully weather this stormy period of their lives.

For Further Thought

1. What physical changes produced the most trauma during your puberty? Why?
2. What insecurities do you have today regarding your body and physical appearance? Why?
3. What preparation did you receive for either menstruation or nocturnal emissions? By whom? Was the preparation adequate?

4. What specific opportunities to build your child's self-esteem are available at this time? Make specific plans to pursue these opportunities.

5. What personal struggles regarding puberty could you relate to your children? How would relating your specific struggles help your children?

6. During adolescence what were you taught regarding masturbation? Did you experience guilt over masturbation? How do you view masturbation now? What advice will you give your child? When would be a good time to discuss masturbation with your child?

7. What item from Dr. Dobson's list do you feel the least prepared to discuss with your child? Which item causes the greatest fear?

Chapter 9

HELP, WE'VE GOT A TEENAGER
(EARLY ADOLESCENCE—AGES 13-15)

Well the last chapter was your basic training. Now you are ready for combat! Many parents dread and fear the approaching teen years, and view the entire time as a massive inconvenience and struggle. However, these potentially troubling years in the life of your child need not be filled with problems and bad experiences. These years can be most rewarding for parents as they help their children navigate the troubled waters and mature into adulthood. I have thoroughly enjoyed the teen years with my children. These years have not been problem free, but we have managed to keep growing and maturing. I challenge you to eagerly anticipate your children's teen years and look forward to a rewarding opportunity to help produce mature, godly adults.

Early adolescence is a relatively new concept in human development. The study of early adolescence has emerged because it is no longer viewed as an unimportant period of development. "Rather, due to increased development and sociological characteristics in individuals, it has become a dynamic, sometimes impacted, growth period which deserves more attention and concern in the future."[1]

Worries, Concerns and Pressures
of Early Adolescence

Adolescence is typically a time of fears, anxieties, and emotional feelings. If you are to have a significant impact on the lives of your adolescents, you must be aware of the primary worries that typify this age. In their book *Five Cries of Parents*, Merton P. and A. Irene Strommen list typical worries of young adolescents, having compiled their information from a survey of over 9,000 adolescents. The worries listed range from the fear that their parents might die to the fear of being beaten up at school.

Many of the worries and anxieties center around physical and sexual concerns such as their looks and their physical development. Dr. Strommen in his survey, asks the question: "How often do you think about sex?" The percentages who said often or very often were:

7th Grade Boys	38%
7th Grade Girls	28%
8th Grade Boys	49%
8th Grade Girls	31%
9th Grade Boys	59%
9th Grade Girls	35%

As these percentages indicate, young adolescents are concerned about sex a great deal of the time. Another related worry concerns the adolescent's feeling of being "in love." Dr. Strommen's research found that 50 percent of early adolescents (grades 7-9) say they are "in love with someone of the opposite sex."[2] It is evident that sex and sexual matters constitute some of the biggest worries and concerns of early adolescents. Add to these normal adolescent sexual concerns the pressures faced by today's teens from the media and our culture's acceptance of sexual liberty, and it quickly becomes apparent that our early adolescent children are under tremendous sexual pressure. Parents need to understand the tremendous pressures on teenagers to have sex. And it appears the pressure works—recent research indicates that 15 percent of seventh graders, 17 percent of eighth graders and 20 percent of ninth graders say they have engaged in sexual intercourse at least once.[3] Parents who are aware of these sexual concerns and anxieties are better able to equip their young teens and help them successfully deal with sexual pressure. Remember, you are the key. By providing information, love, acceptance and nurturing, you will be influencing your young adolescent

---

Most experts agree that rebellion is one of the primary causes of sexual promiscuity and experimentation by early adolescents.

---

tremendously; because according to a 1985 Gallup/AP survey, today's lower-age teens' (ages 13-15) number one desire is for a happy home life.

Dad, Mom and Teen

As they did in the other developmental stages, early adolescents need strong relationships with their parents and positive role modeling from them. From their same sex parents, adolescents need to learn appropriate roles—how to be men or women. And in their relationships with opposite sex parents, they prepare to relate to a future mate. So early adolescence is a time when children need their parents to make time for them and their activities. It is a tragic mistake for parents to believe the myth that teens no longer desire or need to spend time with their parents. While it is true teens are beginning to make strong peer relationships, it is not true that they do not want a relationship with their parents. Rebellious children are usually those who are reacting to poor relationships, either between their parents and themselves, or between the parents themselves. Most experts agree that rebellion is one of the primary causes of sexual promiscuity and experimentation by early adolescents. Some young women even become pregnant just to prove to their parents that they cannot be controlled. So strong family relationships are important and affect many areas of growth and maturity during early adolescence.

Early Physical Development Can Cause Problems
We have briefly discussed problems associated with the early development of certain physical characteristics. Early breast development usually causes girls to become the object of interest and attention from older boys. This is a potentially troublesome aspect of puberty. When young girls begin to receive attention from older boys they are treading dangerous ground. In most cases these older boys are more experienced in terms of boy/girl relationships and can easily persuade younger girls to become more deeply involved in relationships than the girls desire or can maturely handle. For example, young girls may be persuaded by older boys to engage in sexual experimentation, which may lead to all types of sexually promiscuous behavior. Such behavior causes major guilt for a young girl who never intended to become involved in such activity.

Another problem is that girls may learn to relate to males, using their bodies as the primary medium. When this happens, personality development suffers. It appears to them that being successful with boys depends on having a great figure rather than developing personal relationship skills. I have seen young girls learn this lesson well and make it all the way through junior or senior high school using their bodies as the only means of relating to boys. Unfortunately, when social skills are needed later in life, they do not exist. For years I have cautioned parents about the problems associated with allowing early-developing young girls to associate with older boys. I have encouraged parents to watch these girls closely and to regulate their dating and social activities strictly, especially around older boys. This has been a soap-box issue for me because I have seen the damage caused by older boy/younger girl relationships. And on an out-of-town youth activity, I tragically discovered that this issue can also relate to males. A physically mature 14-year-old boy in the group was being treated by older girls as if he were 17 or 18, as his physical appearance might have caused one to believe. This attention was relatively harmless until the boy was approached and enticed into a sexual situation. He was almost forced into sexual activity by a girl five years his elder.

The effect on the boy was devastating, but fortunately he came to me for help. When I discussed this matter with an adolescent psychologist, I was told that such occurrences were increasing. The psychologist told me that the young man would experience the same feelings and emotions as a young girl who had been raped. In my counseling with the young man, this proved to be the case. He felt used, abused and guilty of wrongdoing. The story has a happy ending, however. The psychologist was able to help the young man regain his confidence and deal with his feelings, and today he is doing fine.

But the message to parents is clear. We must constantly be aware of the problems that may be caused by the rapid physical development of our young adolescents, and strictly regulate and monitor their activities, especially those shared with older teens. I recommend that you completely restrict your child from unchaperoned activities involving older teens. In other words, junior high adolescents should not be allowed to "hang out" with high school adolescents on a regular basis. In situations where older and younger teens must be mixed, parents can volunteer to serve as chaperons. The issue is not lack of trust, but simply that young teens do not yet have the maturity to handle potentially damaging situations.

Peer Pressure and Self-esteem

When parents hear the words "peer pressure" they usually cringe. But while it is true that during adolescence, especially early adolescence, peers do greatly influence our children, this influence need not always be negative, and it need not totally replace parental influence. Research indicates that young adolescents are influenced more by their parents than peers. Leah Lefstein of the Center for Early Adolescence at the University of North Carolina says:

> Now you and I know the myth: young teenagers are the victims of tyranny of the peer group. Quite the contrary! Researchers have discovered that young adolescents agree with their parents' views far more often than they disagree. The results of an American study tell us that young adolescents chose to accept the wishes of their parents more often than their peers on 14 of 18 questionnaire items, including church attendance, how late to stay out, opinions of people, and counsel on personal problems. Peers influenced the use of free time, parents were chosen for items involving the development of long-term values.[4]

This is especially true when parents have provided an honest, open and accepting atmosphere during the preteen years. However, peer influence is a major problem with regard to sexual matters, as well as other deviant behavioral areas. A recent Louis Harris Poll found that for both teenage boys and girls, social or peer pressure proves to be the number one reason for premarital sex.[5] Today's teens are under tremendous peer pressure to begin sexual experiences very early. In today's world a very high percentage of teenagers engage in sexual activity. How can we, as parents, offset the negative effects of peer pressure on our children? Let me offer the following suggestions:

1. *Promote a positive self-esteem.* It may seem as if we are overworking this idea, but the importance of a positive self-image cannot be overemphasized. This is especially true when we are talking about peer pressure, because positive, healthy self-esteem gives adolescents the inner strength needed to resist negative peer pressure. When teenagers are caught in difficult situations, a strong sense of identity and a positive feeling of self-esteem will help prevent them

from succumbing to peer pressure. "A young person with a healthy sense of identity will weigh the danger to his or her hard-won feeling of self-esteem against the feelings associated with the loss of peer pressure. When the teenager looks at the situation from this perspective, the choice is easier to make."[6] Unfortunately, the reverse is also true. When adolescents have poor self-esteem for whatever reason, they often gravitate toward any activity that holds the promise of security.

This point was tragically emphasized to me during a counseling session with a teenage girl. She had engaged in sexual intercourse with a young man she really loved, but who apparently was only interested in sex. When I asked her if she had not been afraid she would get pregnant, she said "No, I almost wish I had; then people would know that I had had sex with someone, and they would know that at least one person loved me." This tragic statement is full of lessons for us as parents. This girl comes from a "good Christian home"; yet, somehow she failed to receive the things necessary for a positive self-image. So in her search for acceptance and love, she turned to sex. We have already discussed many ways parents can build self-esteem, and there are many excellent books on the subject which you can consult. Remember, always communicate love, worthiness, and a feeling of competence to your children.

2. *Influence your children by sharing your time.* Our children need to spend time with us. In this hectic world it is easy for parents and children to be insulated from one another. Do not allow this to happen. I have often heard and read about parents who attempt to defend their lack of time spent with their children by saying, "I spend quality time with my kids, even if I cannot spend quantity time with them." This is just a conscience-soothing cop-out. Children need time, period. They need time with parents in order to discover parental beliefs, values and opinions. How can parents hope to offset the effects of peers if they do not spend enough time with their children to impart

their beliefs? David Lewis, a professor and counselor at Abilene Christian University, once said that he had never counseled with a pregnant teenager who had lunch weekly with her father. One way to counteract the influence of peer pressure is simply to spend time with your children and be a positive example for them.

3. *Help your children develop the self-discipline necessary to say no.* The ability to say no is a learned skill. It often takes a great deal of hard work to develop the strength to say no. All people have difficulty saying no in certain situations and areas of their lives. Some of us have difficulty saying no when it comes to overeating, overworking, overspending, and many other areas. Well, parents, imagine your teenager trying to say no to drinking, cheating at school and sexual temptations. My personal experience is similar to that of Dr. Kevin Leman, who says in *Smart Kids, Stupid Choices*, that his experience with teenagers is that "they consciously know that many of the things they do are really not good for them, but they do not have the self-esteem or the self-control to reject them."[7] This is why trite slogans such as "Just say, No!" are overly simple and often do not work. It is one thing to believe you should say no, but quite another thing actually to say no! You must help your children develop self-discipline, which leads to good self-esteem. By teaching responsibility and decision-making, and by allowing the natural consequences of children's actions to occur, parents teach their children that actions have consequences, and that irresponsibility has a price. By learning these lessons, adolescents build their own control mechanisms. They learn not to follow every impulse and to exert self-control, which gives them the strength to say no.

4. *Help your children learn to choose companions carefully.* A normal part of early adolescent development is a movement away from parents and family towards peers. The young person begins looking primarily toward peers for acceptance and confirmation of personal worth. During early

adolescence this transition is made primarily to groups of peers rather than to individual peers. Commitment to individual peers comes during later adolescence. This movement toward peers by adolescents is normal and represents a striving for autonomy and independence. Some teens, however, search for peer acceptance when they have not received approval from their parents. In their search for approval, teens may go along with the standards and behavior of the peer group. As a result, the selection of the peer group assumes tremendous importance. Fortunately, you are not helpless when it comes to whom your adolescent children select for friends. But much of what you can do to encourage your teenagers toward positive peers must be done prior to the early adolescent years and then reinforced throughout these years. People tend to select friends that reflect the image they have of themselves. In other words, adolescents with poor self-images will attempt to find acceptance from others that suffer from the same self-image problem. And teens with strong self-images will have enough confidence to make friendships with people who have good self-images. But, as Dr. G. Keith Olson says:

> This confidence building must begin early and be carried on through the adolescent years. The more effectively parents foster a healthy self-esteem within their children, the greater the chances are that they will seek association with a peer group that reinforces positive growth.[8]

Friendships are important to adolescents, and they need help and encouragement developing them. By welcoming your children's friends, you show your children that you value friendships. Particularly encourage association with peer groups that demonstrate the same basic ideas and beliefs as your family. Parents cannot overemphasize to adolescents the importance of selecting the right friends.

5. *Involve your children in a church youth group.* One way to insure a positive peer influence for your children is to help

them become involved in an active church youth group. When surrounded by peers who share their values, it is much easier for your children to resist negative peer pressure. If the youth group has effective leadership and is structured properly, all young people can find a measure of acceptance and friends who will support, encourage and love them. In fact, I believe that one of the most important functions of a youth group is to provide the kind of support that helps members discover and do God's will. Without such a group of caring Christian peers, youth have great difficulty surviving the stressful years of adolescence.

In the summer months, many youth groups have active programs such as mission trips, camps, outreach and service projects and youth rallies. At the end of the summer I always ask my youth group if it has been harder or easier to resist negative peer pressure during the summer. Almost all of them say it has been easier. When I ask why, they say it's because they spent the entire summer with church friends working toward godly goals. They have been with like-minded people and have experienced the effects of positive peer pressure. Adolescent children need to be a part of an active church youth group—even if it means changing churches.

A Growing Sex-related Problem

Researchers and therapists are reporting a growing problem often related to sexual trauma: the two-sided problem of the eating disorders anorexia and bulimia. Anorexia nervosa is a psychologically-caused aversion to food and a compulsion to be thin. Most anorexics are girls between the ages of 12 and 18. They tend to be perfectionists, and they typically come from middle and upper class families that stress high achievement.

Although there seem to be many causes behind this problem, some therapists report that over 90 percent of the anorexic patients they see have experienced sexual conflict or abuse. Some anorexics may be punishing themselves out of misplaced guilt and shame. Others seem simply to be overly influenced by the constant social pressure in our culture that tells us thin is in and fat is out.

The other side of the eating disorders coin is bulimia—over-eating (binging), often followed by self-induced vomiting and/or excessive use of laxatives (purging). Along with many others under stress, some bulimics seem to resort to over-eating to relieve their anxiety—which, again, often stems from negative sexual experiences. They may then purge themselves of excess food as though rejecting their behavior in disgust. Many people are both anorexic and bulimic, leading to the more recent term "bulirexia." If your teenager shows marked weight changes—either excessive gains or losses—seek professional help immediately!

Why discuss all this here? Obviously just learning the facts about human sexuality is hardly a guarantee against sexual abuse, and resulting problems such as eating disorders. But we discuss it here to underline the fact that children who are brought up with adequate information about sex, communicated in a safe and loving atmosphere, will have a much better chance of overcoming the effects of anxiety resulting from any sex-related problems, including the current virtual epidemic of eating disorders.

Dating

I still remember my daughter's first date—black Saturday! I was too consumed with my own anxiety to be much help with hers. Thankfully her mother was there to calm the fears and anxieties of father and daughter! This parental anxiety is produced by many factors. We begin to realize that our children are growing up and that someday they will leave and get married. It may be caused by memories of our own unpleasant dating experiences. Parents also experience anxiety because they fear they have not prepared their child properly for the dating experience. Dating can stir many emotions and be the source of many family problems and parent/child conflicts.

At the beginning of the dating process parents typically make one of two mistakes. Either they are too restrictive, or they allow dating to begin too early. Overly restrictive parents typically had some negative experiences in their own dating that cause them to overreact and impose unrealistic limits on their teens. Ordinarily these negative or unpleasant experiences were related to their own sexuality. It is important to avoid imposing unrealistic controls and restrictions on teenagers based on our own past mistakes and indiscretions. This only produces conflicts and confrontations with no winners. Evaluate the strengths and weaknesses of your teen and act accordingly, attempting to help make dating a positive experience.

Of all the questions I am asked, one occurs repeatedly: "When should I allow my daughter to date?" I am continually amazed by the number of Christian parents (usually mothers) who encourage early dating or the parents who seem oblivious to the dangers of early dating. The question of when adolescents should start dating is a very serious one and has tremendous sexual implications. There is overwhelming evidence that early dating may lead to early sex. Research done by Brent C. Miller of Utah State University and Terrance O. Olsen of Brigham Young University strongly indicates a relationship between early dating and early sex. Their findings were:

> The younger a girl begins to date, the more likely she is to have sex before graduation from high school. Of girls who begin dating at twelve, 91% had sex before graduation—compared to 56% who dated at thirteen, 53% who dated at fourteen, 40% who dated at fifteen, and 20% who dated at sixteen.[9]

This research also found that adolescents who go steady in the ninth grade are more likely to have sex than adolescents who only date occasionally.

Early dating can affect the sexual habits of adolescents.

Even though many adolescents, especially girls, appear physically mature by age 13 or 14, they actually lack the wisdom, maturity and decision-making abilities to successfully handle one-on-one dating relationships. Since early adolescence is a time teens seek the security of the peer group, it is natural that boy/girl activities should also center around groups. Group activities that involve both sexes seem to be the best beginnings for the dating process. In my church youth group, activities are planned that encourage this group dating. I would strongly urge and recommend that early adolescent

---

Group dating activities will provide the teen with valuable experiences with the opposite sex while at the same time limit one-on-one situations that require greater maturity than most early adolescents possess.

---

youngsters (ages 13-15) be confined to group dating activities. Group dating activities will provide the teen with valuable experiences with the opposite sex while at the same time limit one-on-one situations that require greater maturity than most early adolescents possess. If you choose to allow your early adolescent daughter to begin single dating at age 15 (freshman year), I strongly recommend that she not be allowed to date seniors. There is simply too much disparity between the maturity levels of freshmen and seniors.

When adolescents reach the last half of their sophomore year, or about age 16, they move from early adolescence to late adolescence. At this time most teens are ready to begin single, formal dating. Parents should continue to set limits and guidelines, and going steady should be discouraged.

Limits, Guidelines and Controls for Dating
The beginning of formal single dating is a traumatic time for parents. They suddenly realize how little control they now have over their adolescent. Well before the dating process begins, you should talk to your teenagers concerning certain aspects of this potentially volatile and tempting relationship. The follow-

ing suggestions, when applied to dating, will help your teenagers have healthy, fulfilling dating experiences, which do not involve sexual activity.

1. *Help your teenager set realistic dating guidelines and goals.* The beginning of dating is an exciting and fun time in the life of most teenagers, but because of the potential problems and temptations associated with dating, teens should have certain limits and guidelines. You will need to help your teenagers set realistic guidelines and goals based on their own convictions and beliefs. Notice, I said "help," not "force" or "dictate." Teenagers need to be encouraged to set their own guidelines because parents will not be on dates to "enforce the rules." If the teen is not self-motivated, the standards and rules you have imposed will not work. Parents should set certain basic rules such as curfews and which places are off-limits, but the key here is flexibility.

   For example, assume that you have a rule that your daughter has an 11 o'clock curfew. What if her date to a football game started at eight o'clock and did not conclude until approximately 10:30? Let's say your daughter's date asked her to stop by the local burger barn after the game for a bite. Thirty minutes is not enough time to order, eat, pay the check and drive home. Some flexibility is in order in this situation. Curfews for my daughter were always based upon where she was going, when the event started and ended, and what post event plans involved. And if she ran into time problems she knew to call home. Flexibility and negotiation in the setting of all dating rules help convince teens that their opinions are valued and that they have a part in setting the limits. And when teenagers have participated in the development of guidelines and regulations, they will be far more likely to obey them.

   In addition to guidelines and regulations, teens should be encouraged to think about dating goals. Typically, adolescents who are eagerly anticipating their first date will not think about goals. You should suggest some goals and also have them write their own goals for discussion between you before they begin dating. Some possible goals might include: Why do I want to date? What do I hope to have happen? How can I give and receive acceptance? How do I get to know the other person? How can I have good, clean fun? Helping your teenager internalize a set of realistic goals and standards will launch the dating experience in a fine way.

2. *Encourage your teenager to make specific plans for dates.* Many adolescents do not even know how to plan dates. And many get into sexual trouble because they have not made definite plans for the evening. When counseling with teenagers who have become involved sexually, I always ask when and where the sexual activity took place. Almost always it happened when they were just "messing around." They had no definite plans and as a result there was too much unstructured time. Creative, farsighted date planning helps teens avoid compromising situations. Encourage your teenagers to plan dates in advance, consistent with the guidelines and goals they have set, and keep you informed concerning their plans.

3. *Avoid unchaperoned parties and events.* Unchaperoned parties are not good for teenagers under any circumstances, but they pull in teenagers like a magnet. They are attractive first because no adults are there; second, because there is no structure; and third, because teens can do things they regard as normally reserved for adults such as drinking and having sex. I have very few non-negotiable rules for my children, but one of these rules is: absolutely no unchaperoned parties.

4. *Encourage teenagers to date people who share their convictions.* Whether or not you allow your children to date non-Christians is a private family matter. But I highly recommend that you strongly discourage your children from dating non-Christians. Teens need to understand that they must be careful, not only about their life-style, but also about the life-style of those they date. If teens date others who share their convictions there will be a commitment to encourage and be accountable to each other. However, if the person they

date has lower moral standards than theirs, they may find it easier to compromise their own convictions. Sexual pressures and temptations are difficult to overcome in the best of situations. These pressures are compounded by dating people with different standards and convictions.

5. *Help teenagers discuss sexual temptations, values, and limits openly and frankly.* In discussing sex with teenagers I regularly ask them what are some factors and reasons they have avoided sexual activity. Many teens tell me that one reason they are able to avoid sexual misconduct is because they openly and frankly discuss their temptations, values and limits. Such talks, they say, are held with prospective dates, but not limited to dates. These issues are openly discussed and prayed about by all in the group who share similar values. This is an example of positive peer pressure. These teens help one another by sharing their beliefs, talking about possible temptations, and then holding each other mutually accountable. Of course, it would be inappropriate to begin a relationship with a new friend by completely expressing your sexual temptations and limits, but teenagers need at least some friends with whom they can honestly and frankly discuss these things. Wise parents tell their teens that such disclosure with appropriate people is proper and desirable. They will also make every attempt to see that their teenagers have an environment where such Christian friends are available.

6. *Help teenagers draw the line for their own behavior.* When teens talk about their sexual temptations and values, they need to know in their own minds what their physical limitations are. In other words, in a physical relationship, how far is too far? Is holding hands OK? Is kissing OK? How about French kissing? How about petting and mutual masturbation? Today, sexual standards and expectations vary widely among teenagers.

Teens should be encouraged to set physical limits prior to beginning the dating process. They need to ask themselves "Where is my line, the point beyond which I will not go?"

When this is decided before the situation arises, it proves very helpful.

It is difficult to suggest hard-and-fast rules that apply to everyone. Much depends on the emotional and spiritual maturity of the teen. It is also impractical to assume that teens will not have any physical contact. There will be some kind of touching between a guy and girl as they go through the dating process. But teens need to be encouraged to avoid physical activities that cause sexual arousal to the point of losing control. Sexual arousal is meant to lead to intercourse, and once started, arousal can be extremely difficult to control. In order to avoid losing control, teens need to know their specific limits and avoid people and situations that attempt to stretch these limits. I often tell teens that they can do anything above the neck and below the knees. That simple rule of thumb might not be so bad! Discuss with your teen, prior to dating, specific sexual activities in an attempt to help them "draw the line."

7. *Teach teens they should avoid being alone for long periods of time with their dates.* Teenagers who are serious about setting physical limits will avoid spending large amounts of time alone. A lot of time alone together creates physical opportunities that most teens cannot handle. Parents typically think of sex as taking place in the car, but that accounts for only 6.1 percent of the instances of intercourse between teenagers. Motels and hotels account for another 6.4 percent. Nearly 75 percent of the sexual activity occurs in homes. Twenty-five percent of it occurs in the girl's home, and 51.2 percent occurs in the boy's home.[10] Teens should be cautioned that any situation that could possibly cause them to be tempted should be avoided if possible. In order to avoid these situations and places, teenagers need to think and plan ahead, and need to be keenly aware of their physical limitations. You can help teens escape chancy situations by forbidding them to be at either your or their dates' homes alone. Always make sure you are at home when your teen and a date will be there. It is not enough to have a sibling at

home; at least one parent needs to be present. Also suggest, and request, that after movies and other activities, your teen bring his or her date to your home. A prior agreement between you and your teen can allow for some privacy. Such an agreement helps avoid the likelihood of teens being alone in a car for long periods of time. Also do not be afraid to ask teens where they are going, when they will return and what activities they are planning. To provide real help you need to be involved in the dating process.

8. *Encourage your teen to group date.* Group dating is preferable to single-couple dating because it allows teenagers to be with the opposite sex in a relaxed yet controlled atmosphere. The pressure to become involved sexually is greatly reduced and the absence of this pressure allows them to focus on other aspects of male/female relationships. Too often, teens do not learn to build and develop relationship skills. Group dating provides an excellent opportunity for this. It also exposes teens to a broader spectrum of opposite sex friends. Such exposure to many members of the opposite sex, with multiple relationships and experiences, will help later when they become adults and begin looking for mates.

Many youth ministers encourage group dating. Activities are planned and structured to encourage boys and girls to participate in groups, rather than as couples. For example, in our youth program we never plan activities and say "bring a date." Teens are encouraged to bring a group of friends and, as a service, our older teens with cars invite the underclassmen to ride with them. In group dating boys and girls are free to be themselves and to learn to develop solid opposite-sex relationships.

9. *Discourage going steady.* This is much easier to say than to accomplish, because our society encourages steady boy/girl relationships. Unfortunately, there is a connection between steady dating and sexual activity.

In this context, of course, I am referring to teens who are old enough to car date and who date only one person over an extended time period. I am not alluding to junior high adolescents who repeatedly say they are "going with someone." During junior high "going steady" means that a boy and a girl might speak in the school halls and sit together in the cafeteria. Junior highers change these steady relationships about as often as they change clothes. Junior high relationships should largely be ignored, except if you see a potential problem developing. You should begin in junior high, long before single-dating age, educating and preparing your teens concerning steady dating relationships. Discouraging "going steady" is an uphill battle, but you should create in your teens an awareness of the dangers involved and closely monitor any steady relationships. It is probably impossible to have a teenager pass completely through the dating phase of life and never have an exclusive relationship, but wise parents will continually caution (not nag!) their teens, and carefully oversee and observe their steady relationships in order to detect any troubling signs.

How Do Adolescents Think?

Many parents of early adolescents are so involved in helping their children adjust to all of the physical changes of puberty that often the significant mental changes are often completely overlooked. During early adolescence, or even as early as 11 or 12 years of age, youngsters develop a new thinking process. During the childhood years the thought process is dominated by concrete experiences, observations and facts. During early adolescence the thinking and reasoning process begins to change. Young people move from this concrete period and begin thinking abstractly. They are able to work with symbols and principles, and to develop formal reasoning and propositional thinking. Such new thinking processes allow the adolescent to imagine the future as well as contemplate the past. Dr. G. Keith Olson calls this new thinking process "if .... then." In other words, the teenager can imagine alternatives, anticipate consequences of choices, and systematically reason through problems and decisions.[11]

Often parents erroneously assume that stress, irritability,

anger and sullenness are solely the effects of rapid physical changes during adolescence. But in reality this new way of thinking has opened teenagers eyes to new ways of seeing themselves and others. Their newly discovered thinking process becomes the lens through which their physical bodies and appearance are viewed. This new view of themselves and others, coupled with their abstract thinking ability, enables them to go beyond the real and imagine the ideal. Adolescents often then compare the reality of the world around them to an ideal world of perfection. This idealism, while admirable, causes at least two problems.

First, adolescents just entering this stage become very critical of almost everything in their world—parents, church, society and friends. When criticism is directed toward you as parents, do not take it too seriously, but respond to it in such a way as to communicate to the child that part of growing up is accepting other people. You should also calmly express to teens that you may be equally unhappy with them.

A second problem caused by this new thinking process and critical attitude, is a self-centeredness which generally produces a self-criticism. Teens become consumed by thoughts concerning themselves and their appearance, and they assume everyone else focuses on them as well. They actually believe that when they enter a mall or a school cafeteria all eyes and thoughts are on them. Therefore, they must look and act appropriately or they will be forever embarrassed. When teenagers feel good about their appearance and behavior, they believe that others are also pleased with them. But when teens are filled with self-doubt and self-criticism, they believe others share their negative view of them.

As parents we can best help with egocentric, self-consciousness in our teens by taking a moderate view of things. For example, do not totally accept or reject your teenagers' view of themselves, but try to express your opinion in a positive way that affirms them and at the same time helps them distinguish between their ideal egocentric world and the world of reality. There are other problems related to formal operational thinking in adolescents. These include: having trouble making decisions, argumentativeness, and conflict with family and society. With patience, understanding and love, you can effectively help your early adolescents cope with the trauma caused by their new thinking abilities. Remember that they are as unfamiliar with their new thinking abilities as they are with the rapid physical changes in their bodies.

This newly developed thinking ability provides parents with an excellent opportunity to teach specific lessons about God and His nature to adolescents. Learning about God and His grace, love and forgiveness will help teenagers develop healthy attitudes for the future. Healthy attitudes toward God and His will are crucial for adolescents who are striving to live sexually pure lives because, as we have seen, commitment to God does help many teens avoid sexual activity. I would suggest that parents teach the following spiritual concepts and ideas to their early adolescent children:

1. *It is important to define your values and develop moral standards.* Much trauma during adolescence can be traced to confusion over values and moral standards. This is a time of questioning and offers many opportunities to clarify and strengthen values and standards. Be warned, however, that adolescents do not respond to being told, but they are usually open to being shown! They want to see their parents demonstrate their values and standards rather than merely discuss them. When your life reflects consistency with what you say, then your teen will be more likely to adopt your values and less likely to become confused. Stating values without demonstrating them is ineffective. You need to know what you believe and clearly and explicitly communicate it to your adolescents. It is also a good idea to establish discipline patterns related to values. For example, my children know that I strongly value honesty. And when they have been dishonest or lied I have not interfered or stopped the consequences of their behavior. Values and moral standards are taught and developed when consequences are allowed to discipline children in a natural way. You must also help your adolescents

to use their values in decision making. They must be taught
that good decision making involves asking questions concerning the moral implications of each decision. They must
be taught to evaluate decisions on the basis of what would
be pleasing to God.[12]

2. *God is loving, wise and personal.* In the person of Jesus Christ,
God becomes intimately involved in human life. Jesus was
born and went through puberty and the teen years. He
understands life from our human point of view. Early adolescents need to be made aware of the very personal and
caring nature of God. They need to know that He actually
involves Himself with our problems and is concerned about
all that affects His children. Such a view helps teens begin
developing a personal relationship with a risen Lord. Too
many teenagers are simply taught religious rules and tradi-
tions and when problems and temptations occur there is no
identification with a personal Lord and Savior.

God gave the precious gift of His Son to insure our forgiveness. The death, burial and resurrection of Jesus Christ
confirm the heavenly Father's intention of extending grace
and forgiveness to His children. Jesus Christ is God's living
proof that He is a personal, understanding and forgiving
God. It is crucial for adolescents to understand the spiritual
concept of grace and forgiveness. Adolescence is a time of
many temptations and trials, and most teenagers will be
aware that they have stumbled and fallen short of God's
standards. When failures do occur, however, teens need to
understand that God's grace is unlimited and He forgives
penitent children. It has been my experience that many
teenagers have great difficulty believing and accepting the
grace and forgiveness of God. This is especially difficult
when they have been involved in sexual sins. When parents have practiced and modeled forgiveness in the home,
children have a much easier time understanding and
accepting God's forgiveness. Adolescents need to know that
sins and mistakes are not fatal.

3. *God considers them valuable, important and worthwhile.* Ado-

lescents understand price tags. They generally believe that the higher the price, the more valuable the product. They should be taught that Christians are extremely valuable because of their exorbitant price tag. Christians were purchased with the precious blood of Jesus, therefore, they are of great value. As we have repeatedly said throughout this book, most adolescents suffer from a poor self-image. One way to help our adolescent children achieve a positive self-esteem is to remind them continually that they were purchased with the blood of Jesus, and that God loved them so much that He gave His Son for them.

4. *Through Jesus and the Holy Spirit there is power to overcome sin.* Adolescents need to understand that God has not left His children powerless to defeat temptation and sin. Believers are indwelt by the Holy Spirit and Jesus has promised us help and power in our struggles. Adolescents can be comforted by knowing that God has made provision to help them with their struggles and sins.

5. *Our bodies are sacred and must not be abused.* Early adolescents need to understand that their bodies should be properly cared for because they are sacred trusts from God. Abusing one's body with alcohol, drugs and sex defiles the very temple of God.

6. *God's laws that forbid specific sins, including sexual sins, are for our protection.* Teenagers often see Christianity as merely a list of rules and regulations designed to prohibit their enjoyment and fun. You must communicate that God's laws are for their protection and personal fulfillment. Teens need to be taught that following God's laws and principles insures ultimate happiness and peace. Help your adolescents understand that breaking God's spiritual laws produces unsatisfactory consequences. Often teenagers do not understand this concept because consequences are not always immediate or visible. It is up to you to teach teens the effects of violating God's spiritual laws, and to teach them that ultimate happiness, peace, and personal satisfaction comes from obeying God's laws.

For Further Thought

1. Were you an early or late physical developer during adolescence? Did your rate of development cause trauma? Why?

2. What self-esteem struggles did you have during adolescence?

3. In what area does your adolescent's self-esteem need to be increased?

4. Who are your teenager's best friends? How often are they in your home?

5. At what age did you begin dating? Was your first date a pleasant experience? Were your parents overly restrictive?

6. Have you discussed dating limits and guidelines with your teenager? If not, make specific plans to do so.

7. Make a list of reasonable dating guidelines to share with your teenager.

8. Read 2 Corinthians 6:14-15. How does this Scripture relate to dating?

9. In your opinion, what amount of physical contact is acceptable on dates (holding hands, hugging, kissing, etc.) at your child's present age and stage of development?

10. Did you go steady during adolescence? For how long? Was this steady relationship a positive or a negative experience?

11. Has your adolescent entered the "formal operations" thinking stage? What are some of the signs that have made you aware of this?

12. Has this new thinking process affected your child's spiritual beliefs?

13. Have you discussed your view of God or your theology with your adolescent? If so, does he comprehend your gospel?

14. Plan how you will discuss the six spiritual concepts listed in this chapter with your adolescent.

Chapter 10

THEY'RE ALMOST GONE
(LATE ADOLESCENCE—AGES 16-19)

Some of the topics discussed in the previous chapter anticipated future activities by teens. For example, you were
encouraged to talk with your early adolescents about dating
in order to prepare them adequately in advance for the dating experience. When young people reach late adolescence
they begin in earnest to experience dating and many other
potentially sexual activities. Also, most young people leave
home during late adolescence, so this stage represents a parent's last opportunity for instruction while teens are still in a
somewhat controlled environment. For this reason late adolescence is a very important time for both parent and teen.
We need to discuss several important subjects such as: sex
versus intimacy, how far is too far, a theology of sexuality,
fathers, forgiveness and related topics.

Romance, Love, Sex and Intimacy

Teenagers are greatly influenced by their feelings and emotions, and their decisions are often based on these emotions and feelings. Because adolescents are so emotional they frequently cannot distinguish between romantic feelings, infatuation and love. They believe the romantic notion of a very special person who suddenly appears and sweeps them off their feet. This love-at-first-sight feeling then leads to a perfect relationship that lasts forever. Of course, this myth only works in the movies. In real life there is a big difference between infatuation and true, genuine love.

Intimate relationships are needed and craved by all humans. We desire relationships where understanding, caring, and sharing can take place. And teenagers, with their characteristically low self-esteem, are in particular need of close, intimate relationships. Unfortunately, the confusion between infatuation and real love generally occurs at the same time. The search for intimacy, coupled with an inability to differentiate between infatuation and real love, can lead to sexual involvement by teens. In many instances, sexual activity was not originally planned or desired. A relationship began, based on romantic feelings and infatuation, and continued because of a desire for intimacy. Many young couples who get involved in premarital sex are not really looking for sex; they are searching for intimacy and understanding. When I counsel with teenagers who have become sexually involved, I always ask them what motivated or encouraged them to have sex. Very often at the root of the motivation is a desire for intimacy, affection and love. Sex was not the primary goal. Most adults know that there are differences between sex and intimacy, and that love and sex do not necessarily mean the same thing. But, unfortunately, many teens do not see and perceive these differences.

As parents we have a twofold task: to teach our children how to have intimate, non-sexual relationships and to teach them the difference between infatuation and real love, intimacy and sex. In his book titled *Dating,* Scott Kirby notes the differences between love and infatuation:

1. Infatuation is a feeling; real love involves a commitment also. In real love both the emotions and the will are involved.
2. A person "falls into" infatuation, but "grows into" real love.
3. Infatuation is basically selfish where real love is basically selfless (John 3:16).
4. Infatuation is weakened by time and separation where real love is strengthened by time and separation.[1]

Parents should discuss these differences with their teens in light of the apostle Paul's definition of love in 1 Cor. 13. Adolescents need to understand that real love must be worked at and nurtured continually, and cannot simply be a romantic feeling.

Teaching our children how to have intimate relationships is a lifelong process and probably involves modeling more than teaching. They need to see and understand that it is not only OK to have close, intimate relationships, but it is also necessary for our emotional well-being. When intimacy has been taught and demonstrated throughout the life of a child, it will be easier during adolescence for the child to make distinctions between sex and intimacy. Even when parental modeling and teaching concerning intimacy has occurred, there will continue to be a need to help adolescents clearly see and understand the difference between intimacy and sex. Adolescent girls particularly need to realize that sexual intimacy is not an indication of love. Norman Wright, a noted family and child counselor, in his book *Dating, Waiting and Choosing a Mate*, has a chart that lists some differences between love and sex.

Differences Between Love and Sex[2]

LOVE ...	SEX ...
... is a process; you must go through it to understand what it is.	... is static; you have some idea of what it is like prior to going through it.

... is a learned operation; you must learn what to dothrough first having beenloved and cared for by someone.

... is known naturally; you know instinctively what to do.

... requires constant attention.

... takes no effort.

... experiences slow growth—takes time to develop and evolve.

... is very fast—needs no time to develop.

... is deepened by creative thinking.

... is controlled mostly by feel—that is, responding to stimuli.

... is many small behavior changes that bring about good feelings.

... is one big feeling brought about by one big behavior.

... is an act of will with or without good feelings—sometimes "Don't feel like it."

... is an act of will—you feel like it.

... involves the respect of the person to develop.

... does not require the respect of the person.

... is lots of warm laughter.

... has little or no laughter.

... requires knowing how to thoughtfully interact, to talk, to develop interesting conversations.

... requires little or no talking.

... develops in depth to sustain the relationship, involves much effort, where eventually real happiness is to be found.

... promises permanent relationship but never happens, can't sustain relationship, forever features is an illusion.

Far too many teens are engaging in sexual activity in their search to be loved and understood.

As we teach about love, sex and intimacy and the many differences between these feelings and emotions, it is also an opportune time to teach adolescents that males and females have different views on these matters. For example, there is a large amount of research that indicates that women enjoy hugging, kissing, cuddling, closeness and conversation as much as intercourse. Men, on the other hand, usually associate these activities as merely a warm-up for intercourse. To women, such closeness is an end in itself, to men it is a means to an end. Therefore, intimacy, sex and love can be, and usually are, viewed differently by males and females. An understanding of these differences will provide older teens with a more realistic view of intimacy and sex, and it will also begin preparing them for marriage.

How Far Is Too Far?

We have talked about the importance of discussing dating prior to the actual dating experience. As adolescents begin the dating process, however, there is a need to reiterate the information concerning dating and to address additional dating problems and temptations. This is necessary not only because teens need repetition, but also because it is difficult to understand the nature of the problem or temptation apart from the context of experience. In other words, prior to dating teens will not have a clear understanding of sexual pressures. When actual single dating begins teens will have a suitable context in which to discuss certain problems and temptations. It is particularly important to reintroduce the issue of knowing when to draw the line. Such a discussion raises the question, How far is too far?

As we mentioned previously, it is impractical to assume that teenagers will not have any physical contact. There will be physical touching as teens go through the dating process. In the past couples were warned to avoid petting or physical contact because it might motivate them to "lose control and go all the way." Unfortunately, many teenagers today view matters differently. They "go all the way" without going all the way. That is, they practice some form of mutual masturbation or mutual genital fondling so that an orgasm is reached and sexual gratification is achieved. At the same time they pride themselves on having refrained from intercourse. Sexual experience is gained, but virginity is preserved. This kind of activity is so widespread that a new term has been coined by psychologists and counselors to describe the teens in this category as "technical virgins." They have not technically engaged in sexual intercourse, but they have in fact participated in many sexual activities that result in orgasm. Biblically speaking, they are observing the letter of the law but not its spirit. Since the Bible forbids only sexual intercourse, anything but intercourse is considered fair game (in the teens' minds).

We need to communicate to our adolescents an understanding that being a Christian means obeying the spirit and intent of God's commandments. A quick reading of 1 Thess. 4:3-8 will add another dimension to the discussion. "It is God's will that you should be sanctified: that you should avoid sexual immorality, that each of you should learn to control his own body in a way that is holy and honorable, not in passionate lust like the heathen, who do not know God;...For God did not call us to be impure, but to live a holy life." Teens need to understand that if God did not call us to impurity, He called us to purity. As Christians we are to control our bodies and our lust. Christians are called to "moral purity" which obviously includes more than intercourse.

From a practical standpoint, parents should advise teens how they can avoid going too far. First, advise them never to violate their conscience. Any physical activity that breaches their beliefs or convictions is wrong and should be avoided. Of course, it is possible to train our conscience in such a way that almost anything is acceptable, but godly, spirit-filled teenagers generally know when they are violating their conscience.

Second, counsel them to abstain from any activity that causes sexual arousal. They need to be told that physical sexual activity is progressive. It is designed to progress, ultimately culminating in intercourse. In sex education classes at my church, I draw a graph on the blackboard. I start with hand-holding and proceed through physical activity until reaching sexual intercourse. I then ask the students where they are positioned on the graph. I explain that, whether they agree or not, physical sexual relationships are progressive and that the younger they begin, the faster they will be tempted to progress to the end. Teach your teens that they should avoid arousing situations that will quicken the progression.

Thirdly, teenagers need to be told to avoid touching breasts and genitals. Such touching should not occur either outside or inside clothing. I am constantly amazed by the attitude of many teenagers that touching any part of the body is okay as long as the hands stay on the outside of clothing. The touching of breasts and genitals is extremely arousing and a thin layer of clothing will not diminish this arousal. All touching in these areas should be off-limits.

Fourthly, teens need to be told that often the only way to avoid "going too far" is to end the relationship. This is especially true once sexual activity has taken place. One researcher discovered that "once a pattern of intense sexual relations is established, that pattern is seldom broken except through the termination of the relationship."[3] Christian teenagers who are seriously trying to avoid "going too far" may have to end a relationship.

The question: How far is too far? is an age-old question that causes parents to shudder. In earlier times it was assumed that girls would be less aggressive or would "draw the line" because they bore the brunt of the consequence. Today, however, this is not the case. I, like many others, believed such unaggressive behavior and line-drawing was instinctive. But it now appears that this was a learned or taught behavior. Girls were taught to "draw the line" sexually. As parents, we must teach both our girls and our boys that they must "draw the line" in order to avoid "going too far." They must be taught that even though sexual feelings are very powerful, our God is more powerful, and that a predetermined plan will help to avoid "going too far."

The Gift

During my years of discussing sexual matters with teens I have found a way to approach abstinence and "going too far" that seems to capture their attention. I ask them to imagine finding just the right person and being totally and completely in love with that person. Further they are to imagine that after an engagement the two of them decide to be married. It will be a marriage between two wonderful people who are very much in love. Next I ask them, "What would be the most precious gift you could give that special person? A gift more precious than anything money could buy—a unique gift that is valuable because it is a part of yourself." Then I tell them that the most precious and valuable gift they could give their future loved one is their virginity. It is precious because it is a part of them and can only be given once. And when it has been given, it can never be given again. I explain to them that if they give their virginity to someone else before that special person comes along, they will always regret that this beautiful gift cannot be given to their spouse. This explanation of the specialness and uniqueness of their virginity seems to touch them. Several teens who grew up in our youth program have returned to tell me that this story I call "The Gift" influenced their thinking with regard to premarital sex. Use illustrations, anecdotes, or anything that will help your teens see the importance of their virginity.

Person or Object

In his book, *Growing Up in America—A Sociology of Youth Ministry*, Tony Campolo says:

> Instead of looking at biblical texts that either condemn or affirm sexual activities, it may be more useful to explore how the Bible instructs young people to view these persons with whom they become romantically involved.[4]

In our use-it-and-throw-it-away society, people are often

regarded as objects. If a person is viewed as an object, then that person can be used for personal satisfaction or gratification. But when a person is esteemed as valuable and created in the image of God, abuse is less likely. Teenagers need to be encouraged to understand the value and dignity of all people. They need to learn that by avoiding sexual activity they are displaying respect for themselves and others. Parents should help teens see that as surely as their bodies are the "temple of the Holy Spirit," so also are the bodies of their boyfriends or girlfriends. In other words, parents need to begin at birth teaching the value and dignity of all people and that people are not to

---

Selfish use of others for personal gratification violates the basic message of Christianity.

---

be used as objects. Teaching the value of personhood will have a profound effect on the way teenagers treat members of the opposite sex. Using or manipulating others for sexual gratification will be viewed in a much different light. Any activity that cheapens or diminishes the value, dignity and personhood of others should be avoided. Selfish use of others for personal gratification violates the basic message of Christianity.

Where's Daddy?

Throughout this book I have stressed the importance of the father/daughter relationship. Current research indicates a correlation between the father/daughter relationship and teenage pregnancy. Dr. Grace H. Ketterman, in her book *199 Questions Parents Ask*, says: "In working with a great many teenage pregnancies, I found one of the common denominators of almost all of them was a remoteness from their fathers."[5] Prior to adolescence the mother is generally the major influence in a child's life. But during the teenage years fathers become more influential. Ideally, they offer protection and guidance and demonstrate responsibility. A father's approval and/or disapproval are very powerful factors in a young person's life. He serves as a role model for his son to become a man, and for his daughter's choice of a future spouse. Daughters also gain confidence in themselves as women from experiencing the approval of their fathers. It appears that many teenage girls turn to sexual relationships with boyfriends in an effort to find a substitute for their fathers' love and approval.

During a conversation concerning teenage pregnancy, I asked a caseworker at a home for unwed mothers whether she saw any recurring themes in the experiences of pregnant teens with whom she worked. She immediately responded that during her seven year period as a caseworker almost every teenage girl she questioned said: "I didn't have a very good relationship with my daddy."[6] She further said that a very high percentage of these pregnant girls expressed a strong desire to have spent time with their dads. This does not mean that fathers are completely responsible for their daughters' sexual activity or that a poor father/daughter relationship is totally the fault of the father. However, fathers need to understand their vital role as a major influence in the lives of their teenage girls.

There are several ways fathers can strengthen relationships with their daughters and help prevent pregnancy. First, beginning in infancy, fathers should take an active role in the sex education of their children, including daughters. Many fathers are frightened by the prospect of talking about sex with their daughters, but children need perspectives from both parents, and mothers often resent the fathers' lack of involvement.

Second, fathers should spend as much quality time as possible with their teenage daughters. Fathers who work or play all the time are just the same as gone or dead! Do not assume that your teenage daughter does not need as much of your time as she did as a young child. At this critical age she probably needs more.

Third, fathers should exemplify spiritual leadership. A father's modeling of a Spirit-led life will be a tremendous source of strength and security to a teenage daughter.

Fourth, fathers must be morally pure. I will never forget a conversation with a teenage girl in my youth group. This young lady had very suddenly become sexually active. She was not even attempting to hide her sexual escapades. I asked her to lunch in order to express my concern about the direction of her life. When I asked why she had suddenly turned to sexual activity, her reply was sobering. She said: "My father has been having an affair for two years now, and if he can live like that, then so can I." Obviously the girl was deeply hurt and resentful. She chose to lash out and get even with her father by playing the same sexual game he was playing.

Obviously fathers play an important role with their teenage sons, and mothers influence their teenage daughters, but there is considerable evidence relating to the importance of the father/daughter relationship during the teen years and its effect on teenage pregnancy. Therefore, fathers must very carefully and prayerfully prepare themselves to nurture their daughters through these very difficult years.

Forgiveness

When counseling with Christian teenagers who are either pregnant or have become involved in sexual misconduct, the topic of forgiveness surfaces as a major issue. Premarital sex customarily produces a tremendous amount of guilt. And most Christian teens have difficulty forgiving themselves and receiving God's forgiveness. It has been my experience that the teens who are more easily and quickly able to accept and experience forgiveness have one thing in common—parental forgiveness.

Teens who have been reared in forgiving homes, and who experience genuine forgiveness from parents, heal and recover much more rapidly than teens raised in an unforgiving atmosphere. This point was emphasized to me by a caseworker in a home for unwed mothers. The home housed pregnant teenage girls from many different churches and denominations. The caseworker found that pregnant girls from churches or denominations characterized by a liberating, grace-oriented theology or doctrine, generally chose either adoption or keeping the child, while girls from churches characterized by a more legalistic or restricting theology or doctrine, usually chose abortion. During counseling and questioning the girls who opted for abortion expressed feeling terrified at the thought of talking to their parents about the pregnancy. They did not feel forgiveness was a real possibility.

The pregnancy of your daughter outside marriage or the knowledge that your son is responsible for a pregnancy is one of the most emotionally painful events that can occur in a parent's life. This pain is most intense for Christian parents who, must not only deal with the realities of pregnancy, but who also feel guilt and doubt because their child has apparently rejected their faith and morals. A child's pregnancy affects deeply religious parents in much the same way as the death of the child would. The typical stages of grief are all experienced and healing in many cases takes almost as long as recovering from a loss by death. Christian parents also feel shame and embarrassment when pregnancy occurs. These factors cause some parents to be harsh and unforgiving. But the realities and consequences of the pregnancy are so overwhelming and traumatic that the young people involved do not need the extra emotional stress of unforgiving parents. They need a tremendous amount of love and support. The first step toward helping and healing must be forgiveness. If teens are to choose realistic options and find genuine support, they must experience forgiveness. But in order for forgiveness to occur during such a highly emotional and stressful time, it must be a previously established, routine practice. Begin early in the lives of your children to create a communication system that encourages them to share their sins and failures, as well as their successes. When children are reared in an atmosphere of openness and forgiveness they are better equipped to make difficult decisions, and to determine rationally which options and alternatives are best in a given situation. But unfortunately the opposite is also true—a perceived or real lack of forgiveness confuses teens and interferes with their ability to make intelligent choices.

There are several elements involved in creating an atmosphere of forgiveness. First, parents must forgive themselves. If they have not already sought God's forgiveness for real and specific failures with their teenagers, they should ask forgiveness for busy schedules, overprotectiveness, ill-tempered behavior, or whatever seems to have contributed to problems between themselves and their teens. Once this is done, they need to accept God's forgiveness and continue with the job of rearing their children. Parents need to accept the fact that they will make mistakes with their teens, and that these mistakes can be forgiven and life proceeds. Modeling confession of sins and acceptance of forgiveness also teaches children valuable lessons.

Second, parents must build an atmosphere of forgiveness instead of condemnation. When children, especially teens, are

> Acceptance means allowing a teen to make mistakes and grow from the experience, and then offering needed forgiveness.

constantly criticized and condemned they become excessively guilt ridden. Children who fear criticism, guilt or condemnation, tend to avoid their parents when they have problems or temptations making it impossible for parents to help and support them.

One way parents display forgiveness and acceptance is by not overcorrecting. In their desire to rear successful teenagers many parents spend most of their time and energy correcting. This often causes teens to feel unaccepted. Acceptance means allowing a teen to make mistakes and grow from the experience, and then offering needed forgiveness.

Third, parents can greatly contribute to a forgiving atmosphere by simply saying, "I'm sorry, please forgive me." There is no better way for parents to teach forgiveness than to admit their own mistakes and shortcomings. Parents are sometimes cruel, harsh, forgetful and insensitive. When such failures are openly acknowledged, parents communicate to their children that all people make mistakes and that the way toward healing is to admit mistakes and ask for forgiveness. The simple words, "I'm sorry, I blew it, please forgive me," will teach more about forgiveness than a dozen lectures on the subject.

Fourth, parents must always communicate unconditional love. Children need to know that no action on their part will cause their parents to stop loving them. Unconditional love does not mean that parents can or will remove the consequences of a child's behavior or that some form of discipline will not be necessary. It means that parents will always love the child and will always act in the best interest of the child. When attempting to convey this concept to teenagers I ask them to imagine the worst sin they could possibly commit. Most often teens say that the sin that would hurt, anger and disappoint their parents the most would be becoming pregnant or causing pregnancy.

I then say, "Okay, in the event of pregnancy how would your parents react?" I ask if their parents would throw a suitcase in the middle of the room and say, "Pack up and get out, you are no longer part of this family!" Most teens admit that their parents would not behave so drastically.

I then ask if their parents could remove all the consequences of a pregnancy. I go on to explain that unconditional love means that they will always be a part of their family and that their parents will support, help and encourage them as much as possible, but consequences must still be faced. The central theme of the gospel is this: "While we were still sinners, Christ died for us" (Rom. 5:8). God demonstrates unconditional love and grace toward His children. As parents we must copy God's example.

Expressing forgiveness to young people in this situation is extremely difficult, requiring parents to summon all their inner strength and emotional capabilities. But forgiveness is mandatory, both to heal the teens and to help them make intelligent, rational choices. Do not despair—forgiveness is a gift of God, and when it's needed, He will provide the strength to forgive.

Almost Gone

She has really done it! Our daughter has actually gone off to college and left us. After the final good-byes, as we left the dormitory parking lot, our minds were full of many unanswered questions. Had we taught her enough about life? Was she prepared for college existence? Had we taught and modeled our Christian faith effectively? Was she prepared to handle mature dating relationships? Could she manage money? On and on. Our questions were endless. I had just signed the contract for this book and was (naturally!) thinking about it as well. So I began to question my daughter's preparedness concerning sexual matters. What new or additional sexual temptations would she encounter in her new environment? Thoughts of this kind are especially scary to parents of college freshmen because, for the first time, our teens will be facing sexual temptations without the daily support of their parents and families. But when teens leave home parents have a great opportunity to reiterate many important teachings and principles. They have one last shot to communicate their values and feelings on significant and weighty issues. It has been my experience that because of their greater maturity and the traumatic nature of the occasion, teens are less defensive and better able to discuss important and controversial issues in a rational way. I would advise you to begin talking informally about important topics several months before your teen actually leaves home. The key word is informally. You are not checking off one controversial issue after another, but rather engaging in easygoing conversations to reinforce your child's understanding of your values, beliefs and feelings.

Since our focus is sex education, let me suggest some items that should be addressed before your teen leaves home for the first time.

First, your children should not leave home confused regarding your beliefs on premarital sex and other sexual sins. They should know what you believe and what you believe God's Word says about sexual matters.

Second, as they leave home they should be told that in all likelihood sexual temptations will increase in intensity. Dating relationships after high school are more intense and serious for several reasons including the increased maturity of the teens, greater freedom from interruption and parental controls, and internal and societal pressures on them to marry. Teens should, therefore, be warned that it will take increased effort, dedication and commitment to avoid sexual misconduct now. They also need to understand that they need to become increasingly motivated from within. Hopefully you began teaching responsibility and self-control during the growing-up years, and your teen is now prepared to assume responsibility for controlling his own actions.

A relatively new phenomenon in our culture is "date rape." This term refers to rape that occurs during or after a date with a known, and often trusted, regular boyfriend. The male forces the female to have sex, and simply tells everyone that she willingly agreed. Discuss the possibility of "date rape" with your teenage daughters. This is an excellent opportunity to repeat previously discussed dating guidelines. For example, the admonition to avoid spending great amounts of time alone with a date, and the positive suggestion to group date, would apply when discussing ways to prevent "date rape." Also consider encouraging your daughters to attend a seminar or class in rape prevention, or self-defense, prior to leaving home.

In addition to discussing increased sexual temptation and reemphasizing your values and beliefs, you may consider sharing the experience of your own college years. I am not suggesting that you divulge potentially painful and emotionally damaging secrets or indiscretions, but that you perhaps share some of the struggles and temptations you faced during a similar time in your life. Such sharing will encourage and strengthen teens because they will begin to believe it is possible to defeat temptation, and that mistakes are not fatal and can be overcome with God's help.

Fourth, as teens contemplate leaving home, you should initiate some discussion concerning qualities of a prospective mate. Ask them what specific qualities they are looking for in a mate. In fact, you should start asking this question as teens are entering the last year of high school. It is important for them to be thinking about what is important to them in a future mate, because every person they date is a potential mate. Discuss with your teens the popularly held myth that God has only one special person for them to marry and that if they don't marry that person then a happy marriage is impossible. A marriage involves commitment, hard work and adherence to God's principles for marriage. Therefore, there are many people they could marry and the result would be a happy marriage. Helping teens see this fact frees them to see many possibilities concerning future mates. It also helps them to focus on the real qualities and characteristics of potential mates rather than concentrating on some romantic notion of "the only one."

Fifth, as your teens are leaving home, express confidence in their ability to overcome and triumph over temptation and sin. Your teens, like everybody else, will do much better if they feel others, and especially their parents, believe in them.

Your teen will never be totally prepared to face the world, but do your best and take advantage of this great opportunity to communicate your values, beliefs and feelings once again.

For Further Thought

1. Read I Corinthians 13:4-8. Create an opportunity to discuss with your teen the differences between real love and infatuation.
2. Do men and women disagree about the differences between love and sex? If so, how?
3. Read 1 Thess. 4:3-8. How does verse 4 apply to technical virginity? Write a letter to your teen expressing your beliefs and feelings on this matter.
4. How much importance did you attach to marrying a virgin? Have you discussed your feelings regarding the importance of virginity with your teenager?
5. Fathers, when was the last time you had a "date" with your daughter? Make a "date" for this week.
6. Complete the following: When I think about my role as a parent, I have difficulty forgiving myself for....
7. When was the last time you said "I'm sorry" to your child? What behavior precipitated this statement?
8. If your teenager was leaving home today and you could tell her/him only three things, what would they be?

Chapter 11

ADDITIONAL DIFFICULT TOPICS

I have saved several topics until the end of the book. This does not mean I am inferring that these subjects should not be dealt with until after teens reach or pass older adolescence. Like most of the information in this book these topics should be discussed with children whenever they express an interest or need to know the information. As we have repeatedly stated, sex education is an ongoing, lifelong process, so you should be prepared to have frequent talks about all areas of human sexuality, especially about highly emotional and controversial topics such as sexually transmitted disease (STD), birth control, abortion and homosexuality. It would be extremely difficult for parents to explain all of their beliefs and feelings on any of these subjects in one or two attempts. It is also very difficult in a book such as this to cover all the issues related to these sensitive subjects. Our focus will be on helping you present rational, biblical viewpoints to your teenagers.

Sexually Transmitted Diseases (STD)

Some subjects in life are so unpleasant or disgusting that we often simply ignore or avoid even the mere mention of them. One such topic is venereal disease. This subject is so frightening and offensive that most people simply pretend it does not exist, and they are therefore woefully ignorant about this ugly area of human sexuality. In *Raising a Child Conservatively in a Sexually Permissive World,* Sol Gordon lists some popularly held myths concerning these diseases:

1. Syphilis and gonorrhea are the only serious venereal diseases in the United States.
2. STD can be transmitted only by genital contact.
3. Once the signs of STD disappear, the person is cured.
4. Once you contact STD you certainly know you have it.[1]

Such myths prove how uninformed many of us are concerning sexually transmitted diseases. Our object in this section of the book is to inform you about these diseases and help you pass this information to your teens. Let's begin by looking at some statistics regarding sexually transmitted diseases:

- Every day 33,000 Americans become infected with a sexually transmitted disease.[2]
- The American Social Health Association estimated in a 1980 report that from 5 to 20 million Americans have herpes. The number is growing at a rate of approximately 500,000 cases per year.[3]
- Physicians now are familiar with about 25 different diseases that are transmitted through sexual contact, which together cost the public over 2 billion dollars annually in health care.[4] Of these, at least five must be reported to the Department of Health by your doctor because they are so hazardous to health and are highly contagious. The five are: syphilis, gonorrhea, chancroid,

granuloma inguinal, lymphogranuloma.
• STD now constitutes the number one reportable communicable disease in the United States. The problem is most serious among young adults, where the STD rate in the 16 to 20 age group is three times the level of the general population. In 1981 the greatest increase in gonorrhea cases was among youngsters 10 to 14 years of age.[5]

As the above statistics attest, sexually transmitted diseases have reached epidemic proportions in this country. There are several possible reasons for this epidemic, including increased sexual promiscuity, ignorance and professional and public apathy. Whatever the reasons, these statistics are shocking.

It is important to inform your early adolescents about sexually transmitted diseases and discuss the subject thoroughly. This kind of informational discussion is not based on the assumption that your teens will be sexually active. It is rather based on the belief that adequate knowledge will promote responsible behavior and encourage abstinence. When you provide this information during early adolescence, your teen will have additional facts on which to base decisions. Unfortunately, teenagers make mistakes and lose control of themselves. If sexual activity does occur, there is always the risk of STD. Ignorance of the facts concerning STD will only compound an already painful situation. So prepare your adolescents adequately with regard to STD. Hopefully, they will never need the information personally, but if the need arises, adequate STD information may save their lives.

In general, adolescents need to know that some forms of STD are highly contagious. They also need to know that the term STD refers to infections that can be transmitted during intimate body contact other than sexual intercourse. In other words, STDs are diseases that are capable of being transmitted through contact with the genitals, the anus, the mouth and other body areas. You may be thinking that such information will unnecessarily scare your teenagers. There are two points I want to make in that regard. First, awareness of the dreadful consequences of sexually transmitted diseases may save their lives, so let them have some fear. And, secondly, if being scared of sexually transmitted diseases aids teenagers in avoiding sexual misconduct and in remaining pure as God intended, then a little realistic fear has done its work.

Parents and teenagers should be aware of the signs of STDs. In general, a woman should seek medical help if she has any of the following signs.

- Burning while urinating.
- A persistent sore throat.
- Pain or itchiness in or around the vagina.
- Any soreness or redness around the vulva or the anus.
- Any sores, warts or pimples in or near the vulva.
- A discharge that is yellow, green or otherwise discolored. (A normal discharge is usually clear or milky.)
- A thick discharge that looks like cottage cheese.

In general, a man should seek medical help if he has any of the following signs:

- A persistent sore throat.
- Burning during and shortly after urination.
- Any sores, warts or pimples on or around the penis.
- Any unusual coloring of the urine, such as urine which is reddish or very dark.
- A milky or puslike discharge.
- Any soreness or redness around the anus.[6]

For information concerning specific sexually transmitted diseases, consult a physician. Specific information can also be obtained by writing the American Foundation for the Prevention of Venereal Disease, Inc., 799 Broadway, Suite 638, New York, NY 10003.

AIDS

By far the most frightening sexually transmitted disease is AIDS. The AIDS virus attacks the body's immune system, dangerously lowering resistance and producing a condition in which the body cannot protect itself against disease. The body becomes highly susceptible to pneumonia and other contagious illnesses. In 1988 there were approximately 54,000 diagnosed AIDS cases in the United States, with reported deaths of almost 31,000 people.[7] And according to former United States Surgeon General, C. Everett Koop: "By the end of 1991, an estimated 270,000 cases of AIDS will have occurred with 179,000 deaths in the United States."[8] And in addition to these diagnosed cases, an estimated 1.5 million to 2 million people in the U.S. are carriers of the AIDS virus. Ninety percent of these carriers are unaware of their condition.[9]

AIDS presents a rather bleak picture. Many people have questions regarding its origin, because up to about 10 years ago, AIDS was unknown in the United States. The question is asked, Why has it not been around for centuries? since AIDS is primarily regarded as a disease associated with homosexuality, and at least 10 of the first 14 Roman Emperors were homosexuals. The best scientific research indicates that AIDS is a new virus that originated in Africa. Scientists believe that it was probably transmitted to man from monkeys. Either the monkeys bit humans, or humans drank monkey blood or ate monkey flesh. Once the virus was in humans it behaved differently than any previously known disease. This new disease gained a foothold in Africa during the late '60s; it then was carried to Haiti in the '70s, and to the United States in the early '80s. The disease is much more prevalent in Africa. Some researchers believe that as many as 10 million people on the African continent now have AIDS, and that in the next 10 years tens of millions of Africans will die of AIDS. In Africa, the ratio of AIDS cases is one to one among males and females. In the United States, the ratio is five to one, the majority being males.[10]

Most people associate AIDS with homosexuality, but the disease is spreading rapidly among heterosexuals. Most AIDS victims, however, are from the following high-risk categories: sexually active homosexual and bisexual males, intravenous drug users, people who receive blood transfusions, infected mothers, and sex partners of the above.

In light of the frightening and dangerous nature of AIDS, it is important that adolescents be thoroughly informed concerning this dreaded disease. I believe parents should furnish their adolescent children with factual and accurate information regarding all aspects of this disease. In transmitting these facts to your children, dispel the myths and make certain they

---

Information concerning AIDS, as well as other STDs, should be furnished to teenagers.

---

understand the life-threatening possibilities of this disease. You should tell your adolescents the following about AIDS:

1. The AIDS virus is present in, and can be transmitted through body fluids or discharges such as blood, semen, and vaginal secretions.
2. Rectal, oral and vaginal sex can transmit AIDS. It can be transmitted from a man to a woman, or a woman to a man during heterosexual intercourse.
3. There is a one in 85 chance that vaginal sex will transmit AIDS. Ten percent of AIDS victims contracted the disease through heterosexual sex.
4. As it relates to AIDS, sexual intercourse involves not only the current partner, but also everyone with whom the partner has had sex for the past several years.
5. There have been no confirmed AIDS cases as a result of: kissing, sneezing, coughing, hugging, sharing food, mosquito bites, masturbation or using toilet seats.
6. It is possible to contact AIDS from someone who

is unaware they have the disease, because it is possible to have the disease, or be a carrier, without experiencing symptoms.

7. Condoms are only about 80 percent effective in preventing AIDS—that means there is a 20 percent risk.

8. The best way to prevent AIDS is to remain sexually pure until marriage. Abstinence offers the only sure protection against AIDS.

Information concerning AIDS, as well as other STDs, should be furnished to teenagers. The purpose of sharing this information is to equip them with relevant, factual knowledge related to sexually transmitted diseases. This knowledge and information will assist them in making sound decisions. And, by sound decisions I mean the total avoidance of sexual activity until marriage.

Birth Control

A highly controversial aspect of sex education relates to teaching about birth control. This subject is especially emotional for Christian parents because sometimes parents cannot tolerate the idea that their own teenagers might have sexual relationships. Even Christian parents should be aware that 50 percent of high school girls have sexual intercourse before graduation; this is an inescapable fact of the world in which we live. Therefore, the much debated question is, should adolescents be given information concerning birth control? And, is the simple giving of knowledge interpreted by adolescents as permission to be promiscuous and participate in sexual activity? These are not easy questions to answer, but as parents we need to understand that the stakes are high. "Research reveals that less than 20% of sexually active teenagers use contraception of any form the first time they have sex. Only 30% use some reliable form of contraception as they continue to have sexual intercourse."[11]

The facts clearly indicate that record numbers of teens are having sexual intercourse. Similarly, it is clear that most sexually active teenagers do not use any form of birth control. When pregnancy inevitably occurs, these same teens turn to abortion as the easy escape. Perhaps we should begin our discussion with an analysis of the reasons why teens do not use birth control. This will help you gain a better understanding of the adolescent mind. And hopefully this understanding will equip you to handle discussions on this very difficult subject.

There are several reasons why teenagers do not use contraceptives. First, as I have mentioned several times, many teenagers suffer from a very low self-esteem. Girls in this situation often actually want to get pregnant. They feel alienated and unloved by the significant people in their lives, and they fantasize that a baby will fill the void and make them feel loved and useful. So, in order to fulfill this fantasy they do not use birth control. In younger adolescents, rebellion is a major reason for pregnancy. These young girls are using pregnancy as a way to rebel against their parents and assert control over their own lives They want to get pregnant as a way of rebelling.

Another reason teenagers do not use contraceptives relates to what several adolescent experts refer to as the "personal fable." This fable is very prominent during adolescence and revolves around the teenager's belief that he or she is unique and special and as a result of this specialness is shielded by a cloak of invulnerability. In other words, they believe that bad life situations such as cancer, auto accidents, and even death, do not happen to them. This belief in a personal fable leads teens to conclude that pregnancy cannot happen to them.[12] Therefore, they do not use contraceptives because, after all, their uniqueness protects them from life's problems.

Perhaps the primary reason teenagers, especially Christian teens, do not use birth control is that it would make sexual intercourse seem premeditated. In other words, the use of birth control would indicate a prior plan to sin or to go against God's laws. In the teen's mind, if sexual intercourse occurs during a highly passionate moment of uncontrolled emotions and feelings, the act does not produce as much guilt. On the other hand, if contraceptives are purchased and their use planned, more guilt is produced because it is impossible to blame unrestrained passion. So they deny and do not accept responsibility for becoming sexually active. They claim some innocence by saying, "It just happened."

Hopefully a lifetime of teaching children that they are sexual beings and that they need to control physical cravings will help prevent sexual activity from "just happening." From their earliest years children should be taught that actions have consequences, and that people take precautionary measures to avert damaging situations. A lifetime of this kind of teaching will help avoid accidents.

But, back to our original question: Should adolescents be given information and knowledge concerning birth control, and does such knowledge, if provided, encourage or promote promiscuity? Obviously, these questions are very controversial and there are no easy or correct answers, only opinions. Basically there are two schools of thought on this issue. Some people believe that by providing adolescents with information and knowledge concerning contraceptives and birth control, we are encouraging them, and even giving them permission, to have sexual intercourse. These people theorize that if adolescents are unaware of factual knowledge concerning contraceptives, they will not be sexually active. Other people believe that parents are responsible for teaching teenagers how to avoid pregnancy, and that teens should be furnished information related to contraceptives and birth control.

The birth control issue is so highly charged emotionally that people on each side of the question often make false assumptions concerning those on the other side. For example, people who oppose teaching about birth control, traditionally believe that the advocates of such teaching are opposed to teaching abstinence. And those people who propose teaching about birth control, accuse the opponents of being unrealistic and shortsighted. But I believe it is possible to teach about sex and promote abstinence, while at the same time maintaining a realistic view of teenage sexual conduct, and providing factual knowledge concerning birth control. I do not believe it must be an either/or proposition. "Youngsters can make sharp distinctions between knowing and doing; between factualism and propriety; between what is possible and what is right for them."[13]

I would suggest that parents not dilute their own and God's view on sexual sins. Sex before marriage remains a sin. You should clearly communicate this fact to your teens. But, I also feel that teenagers can be told that, if they choose to violate parental and godly views, they should protect themselves and use contraceptives. One researcher says:

> Another approach is for parents to say, "Look, we don't want you to have sex, but if you are going to anyway, we want you to use birth control." This is not a double message. It clearly states the parent's feelings, but it also says that if the children choose not to obey (a realistic possibility) they still have a duty to act responsibly.[14]

During the past several years I have interviewed many Christian psychologists and counselors. I have also researched the writings of many professional psychologists, counselors and sex therapists. I have not been able to find any evidence that providing birth control information to teenagers encourages sexual activity. And many of these people have done extensive research on this subject. In a telephone interview, Dr. Ron Rose, a family therapist, stated:

> I have not seen any scientifically done research indicating that the giving of information and knowledge concerning birth control, promotes sexual activity. In fact, most research indicates the opposite.

My own experience, while not of a scientific nature, confirms these findings. For 10 years I have talked with teenagers in my youth group on this subject. During sex education classes and discussions I have said something like this: "Sex before marriage is damaging and sinful. It should be avoided at all costs. But if you choose to disobey God and your parents, then you should protect yourself and use some form of birth control." In subsequent private conferences I have asked numerous teenagers, including my own children, if they interpreted my remarks as giving permission to have sex. I have yet to have one girl or boy answer yes! You see, for many years these teens have been taught by me that sex before marriage is wrong, and a few informational remarks regarding birth control cannot possibly undo all that prior teaching. It will be the same with your children. When your lifelong message is one of sexual abstinence before marriage, your children will not misinterpret your feelings. And for those few teenagers who directly disobey God and parents, at least they will be spared additional problems.

I am not advocating the distribution of contraceptives, merely the giving of knowledge and information. Knowledge is neither moral nor immoral. Christian teenagers engage in sexual activity because they have low self-esteem, because they have poor relationships, either at home or with their peers, or because they have allowed themselves to be in a situation where physical contact is extremely difficult to control and they have succumbed to temptation. But I have never read, heard or seen any evidence that Christian teenagers have had sexual intercourse because they had a knowledge of birth control or because it was available.

Abortion

Abortion is one of today's most controversial and hotly contested social and political issues. It affects not only adults, but also teenagers. People are militant on both sides of this issue, and a stance of logic and reason is hard to find and keep. Space does not permit an in-depth discussion of all the details and ramifications of this highly emotional and controversial subject. I am speaking from the position of a Bible-believing Christian, who is opposed to abortion. (Some Christians do believe in abortion when the mother's life is in danger or when rape has occurred.) Our discussion will focus on what our teenagers should be told about abortion and/or possible alternatives for dealing with teenage pregnancy.

Some parents believe abortion should not be discussed because to discuss the subject would be to admit the possibility of pregnancy. Once again the fallacy is the belief that knowledge, in and of itself, is harmful. But a clear statement of beliefs concerning this important topic will help our teens make intelligent, godly decisions. Hopefully, our teens will avoid pregnancy altogether. But if that is not the case, they need clear, accurate information regarding choices available to them.

A teenage girl has four choices when pregnancy occurs: give the baby up for adoption, marry the father of the child, raise the child alone or have an abortion. Regardless of her choice, she will probably have to make it alone, since research indicates that more than 85 percent of boys who impregnate teenage girls eventually abandon them. Abortion is often seen by the teenage couple as the most efficient and least troublesome choice. It requires no marriage and appears to allow all parties to resume normal life-styles after a quick, simple, medical procedure. It sounds neat, clean and easy. To immature, troubled teens, abortion resolves the situation for the moment. However, teens need to he told about the terrible emotional problems abortion often causes in girls and women. The guilt often continues for years. One researcher found that long-term stress related to abortion continued for up to 10 years after the abortion, with more than half the women suffering from nightmares related to the abortion. My own experience, while limited, confirms this.

All of the women I have talked to regarding their abortions, have expressed deep regret or guilt. Several of these women have accepted God's forgiveness and resumed a productive Christian life. Others have been devastated by the abortion experience. Even the well functioning women, who have accepted forgiveness, have some guilt and regret. They indicate that there will always be the burning question, What would my child have been, or done? Teenagers need to be told that abortion is not as simple or as easily and quickly forgotten as they might think. Guilt can be a devastating emotion, especially when spread over an entire lifetime.

During many years of youth work I have had several opportunities to minister to pregnant teenagers and their families. One surprising aspect of this ministry relates to abortion. I have been astonished at how quickly Christian parents view abortion as an alternative. This is especially true when parents first discover that their daughter is pregnant. One of my coun-

All people should be treated with dignity. This applies to the born, as well as to the unborn.

seling talks with these families is to convince them that abortion is not a good choice. It should be pointed out that the families I am referring to are Christian families who were totally and completely opposed to abortion before the pregnancy of their daughters. When abortion could be viewed simply as theory or a problem of others, abortion was opposed. But when the theory became their reality, different viewpoints surfaced. I should also point out that, in most cases, I and others were able to persuade these families against abortion. My point is this—whether in relation to abortion, other sexual matters or life in general—children must see consistency between what parents say during the calm and what they do during the storm. When parents say one thing and then attempt to do something altogether different when difficulties arise, children receive double messages. These double messages cause confusion about right and wrong.

I believe there are two attitudes that parents can begin teaching and demonstrating early in the life of their children that will create an atmosphere in the home that will greatly discourage abortion. First, parents should create and maintain a forgiving system with their children, one that encourages them to admit and share their sins, mistakes and failures. We have talked about the importance of forgiveness and its relevance to abortion. Many religious, church-going teens choose abortion because they conclude that forgiveness is impossible and they opt for the quick fix. Children reared in homes where the forgiveness of Jesus is taught and modeled can better review all options and make decisions based upon the interests of the unborn baby instead of their own guilt. A forgiving atmosphere is vital in the prevention of abortion.

In addition to a forgiving atmosphere, children should be taught the sanctity of all life. Help your children understand that life is a gift from God and therefore very precious. Human life, especially, is holy because we are made in the image of God. We teach our children about the sanctity of life by valuing and respecting all people and by avoiding racism, sexism and any other "isms" that devalue or degrade human life. All people should be treated with dignity. This applies to the born, as well as to the unborn. Abortion violates the sanctity of life by killing the unborn, but as Christians we must be concerned about the sacredness and dignity of the born as well. We must teach our children to show concern, compassion and kindness to all human life—born and unborn—and exemplify the compassion of Jesus to all humans. When children have been taught to view all life as a precious gift of God and that, as such, it has sanctity and holiness, then they will be much less likely to view abortion as a viable solution.

Christian individuals and churches alike must do more than condemn abortion.

> Churches and other groups opposed to abortion must be prepared to extend practical help to both the unmarried woman who is pregnant, and the married woman who may be faced with the question of abortion. Merely to say to either one, "You should not have an abortion," without being ready to involve ourselves in the problem, is another way of being inhuman.
>
> The unmarried woman may need a place to stay.

Time should be taken to tell her about the many couples who cannot have babies who long to have a child to adopt. She will certainly need counsel about how to care for her child if she decides to keep the baby. Pleasant institutions should be available for unmarried women awaiting the birth of a baby, but each person who does not believe that abortion is right should personally be prepared to offer hospitality, financial aid, or other assistance.[15]

In communicating your beliefs concerning abortion to your teens, the procedure itself and its emotional trauma should be portrayed realistically. It is important that teens comprehend exactly what it means to have an abortion. In addition, you should help them positively to explore all the other options available to them.

Homosexuality

For Christians, few issues cause more intense emotional feelings and reactions than the topic of homosexuality. Fear is among the most common reactions to this behavior. Parents fear that their children might become homosexual, and teenage boys fear that they might be gay.

Simply defined, homosexuality means preferring or choosing to pursue sexual gratification with members of the same sex. However, in real life, defining homosexuality can be far more complicated, and simplified definitions often cause problems. For example, many adolescent and preadolescent boys have numerous fears regarding homosexuality. They worry about being or becoming homosexual because of involvement in sex play or mutual sexual exploration. Some sex play is normal for boys of this age and most fears regarding homosexuality are completely unfounded. You should relieve this anxiety for your adolescents by informing them that sex play happens commonly and generally has no relationship to future sexual identity.

The cause or causes of homosexuality have been hotly

debated in both Christian and secular circles for many years. Opinions and theories span the spectrum. Some people view homosexuality as a terrible sin and as appalling behavior practiced by depraved individuals. Others believe it results from a genetic or hormonal malfunction. Still others believe homosexuality is primarily a learned behavior acquired as a result of a dysfunctional family. Attempts to understand homosexuality and its causes are difficult because of emotionalism, distortion and debate regarding interpretation of scientific and psychological data. In addition, great disagreement exists among leading experts in the fields of science, medicine, psychology and religion.

In spite of the absence of a consensus of opinion on the causes of homosexuality, however, a more detailed examination of these causes will be helpful to parents. Following are four of the more frequently cited causes of homosexuality.

Genetic inheritance or predisposition

"Contemporary researchers and theorists do not believe that homosexuality is inherited. Some of them believe, however, that certain people inherit a propensity toward same sex or bisexual traits and preferences."[16] Of course, such a theory is very controversial and often considered heretical among Christian people, and many overreact and fail to understand what such a theory suggests. Most proponents of this theory are saying that a genetic condition may predispose a person to same-sex preference. "This does not mean that all persons so predisposed become homosexuals, only that they may be more likely to learn same-sex preference."[17] This theory should not alarm Christian people because, even if it is valid, having a predisposition does not guarantee that the person will become a homosexual. This would only take place as the result of conscious choices made later in life.

Negative parental or family influence

Many researchers and psychologists believe homosexuality is a learned, or acquired, response produced as a result of a dysfunctional family. In other words, families, especially parents, can greatly contribute to homosexual behavior. Fathers who are unaccepting, detached, cruel, angry or passive are more likely to produce children with homosexual tendencies. Mothers who are overprotective, threateningly powerful, dominant, possessive, permissive and overly critical are likely to produce the same results. The combination of a parent who acts in a powerful, dominant and controlling manner with one who appears passive, incompetent and scared, creates a climate very conducive to developing homosexual tendencies in children. Ideally, children need to learn the qualities and characteristics of males and females from their parents in a noncompetitive atmosphere where the parents accept, respect and love each other. Children need to spend a good deal of time with their same sex parent. The opposite sex parent should encourage and approve such expenditures of time. Dads should be teaching sons, and mothers teaching their daughters. Psychologists and therapists rarely see homosexuals who report good relationships with their fathers, in which plenty of time was spent together.

Seductive childhood experiences
Many children have encounters with older homosexuals (although the incidence is probably lower than cases of heterosexual seduction). While such experiences certainly do not automatically turn young people into homosexuals, encounters of this nature do seem to have played a significant role in the lives of many homosexuals. This kind of seduction can influence children toward homosexual habits before they are old enough to understand properly what is happening.

Loss of sexual role models and definitions
In today's society many children have no role model in the home. Divorce contributes to this loss of role models in many homes, and children from single parent homes are believed by some to be at higher risk regarding their sexual identity. Another theory regarding homosexuality concerns the loss of sexual role definition in today's world. In times past there were clearly distinguishable differences between men and women.

The sexes looked, dressed and acted in discernibly different ways. Today, hairstyles, fashions, jobs, attitudes and behavior are so similar that differences between males and females are blurred. In some ways this is good for society, but for children struggling with sexual identity, today's unisex habits can be extremely confusing.

There are many other theories concerning the causes of homosexuality but most professionals agree that there is no single cause; it is a multifaceted problem.

A friend of mine who is a clinical psychologist reported to me that the success rate for curing homosexuals was only about 10 percent. I cannot authenticate his figures, but my research does suggest that most professionals believe curing homosexuality is very difficult. However, there are things parents can do to reduce the likelihood of homosexuality becoming the preference of their children.

1. *Maintain good healthy attitudes toward males and females.* Negative, critical attitudes aimed at an entire sex can cause children to reject themselves as part of a whole gender. Parents of both sexes must accept maleness and femaleness and project positive attitudes toward both sexes. Such acceptance helps children understand and accept their maleness or femaleness. Children reared in homes where positive attitudes toward both sexes are taught and demonstrated, usually have healthy sexual identities.

2. *Protect young children.* Furnishing young children with gruesome details about homosexuality can confuse and frighten them. However, children must be protected from the many dangerous influences in today's world. We have talked about preventing molestation, and I gave several suggestions to help children avoid dangerous situations. If younger children have been properly trained to avoid unfamiliar situations and people, they will have no need of explicit information regarding homosexuals. Graphic descriptions of any kind of sexual abuse should be shunned. The pivotal issue in protecting young children is being aware of potentially harmful circumstances or situa-

tions. For example, you should be well-acquainted with baby-sitters, nursery attendants, neighborhood parents and all other persons with whom your children might have unsupervised contact. If you have any doubts or suspicions, keep your children away from the person in question. Unfortunately our world is not always a nice place, and the protection of our children demands high parental visibility.

3. *Encourage teenagers to avoid certain situations.* Teenagers should be helped to avoid situations where temptations may arise. As we have discussed earlier, many teens are easily confused when they engage in normal same-sex play. They fear the experimentation may cause them to become homosexual. In addition to relieving their fears, you should suggest ways for teens to avoid tempting situations. For example, when friends stay the night suggest that they not sleep together. Also in your discussions with them regarding masturbation, you should tell them that even if they occasionally feel the need to masturbate, under no circumstances should it be done in the presence of others. In addition, encourage them to report immediately to you any time they are propositioned by someone of either sex. Temptations avoided are temptations defeated.

4. *Teach God's model for the family.* Begin early in your children's lives teaching God's model for families. God created a system of monogamous sexual union between a man and a woman. God intended sex to be heterosexual and confined to marriage. Children need God's concept of marriage and sex constantly taught and demonstrated in their presence. One counselor put it this way:

> I have never seen a homosexual come from a home where both mother and father were incurably in love with Jesus Christ and with each other.[18]

5. *Parents must be effective role models.* In order to demonstrate properly how an adult of your sex acts, you must spend time generously with your children. You may be thinking at this point that I have a one-track mind because over and

over again I have advised and encouraged parents to spend time with their kids. But I know of no other way to teach and train children effectively apart from time invested in them. Little boys will learn to be men only by observing and doing. Girls become women by watching and engaging in activities with their mothers. To develop healthy sexual identities children must spend time with same sex parents. And time spent with opposite sex parents helps children appreciate and accept the other sex. Effective parental role modeling is a crucial factor in the prevention of homosexuality.

6. *Promote sex role differentiation.* You must teach against chauvinism, sexism and other negative attitudes toward the opposite sex. But children also need healthy feelings concerning their own masculinity or femininity. Encourage pride and acceptance in your child's sex. Both sexes are uniquely designed by God, and children need proud, positive attitudes regarding their own sex. You help to promote such attitudes in your children by accepting them and by discouraging society's unisex attempts to remove the distinctions between men and women. Men and women are truly equal, but they are also very different. Our children need to learn this lesson.

Preventing homosexuality, like preventing other forms of sin, involves a lifetime of teaching and modeling. Hopefully you will find the suggestions I have given to be helpful and beneficial. But please remember to seek God's guidance often when confronting these difficult parenting tasks.

Most people, including many Christians, have a strong aversion to homosexuals. This extreme repugnance causes many to develop what some psychologists and counselors are calling "homophobia"—fear of homosexuality. And, unfortunately, many Christians do not attempt to help homosexuals, but instead completely reject them and view this sin as being the worst possible sin. Parents often reject their own children because of homophobia. Such intense feelings raise two very important questions: What specifically does the Bible say about homosexuality, and how should Christians treat homosexuals?

There are references to homosexuality in both the Old and New Testaments (Gen. 19:1-10; Lev. 18:22; 20:13; Rom. 1:25-27; 1 Cor. 6:9-11). While God's Word does not dwell at length on homosexual behavior and does not seem to regard it as worse than other sins, the Bible does plainly judge homosexuality as sin. The Bible also clearly condemns heterosexual intercourse outside of marriage. So homosexual acts as well as heterosexual acts outside of marriage are both sin. But fleeting sexual thoughts of any kind are not sin unless dwelt on to the point of fantasy, at which time they become sin. All sexual lusts, fantasies and acts are sinful when practiced outside God's plan.

My point is simply this: Practicing homosexuality is sin, but the homosexual should be treated in the same way as any other person who commits sin. Our response ought to be exactly the same as toward any other sinner. A Christian response to homosexuals should not be fear and critical judgment (homophobia). We should attempt through love and kindness to persuade homosexuals to accept redemption by the blood of Jesus. In 1 Cor. 6:9-10, homosexuality is listed with a group of other sins, and it goes on to say that such people will not inherit the kingdom of God. But in verse 11 we read: "And that is what some of you were. But you were washed, you were sanctified, you were justified in the name of the Lord Jesus Christ." The homosexual's only hope rests in the grace, forgiveness and Lordship of Jesus. A cure will also involve good professional counseling, and a desire to be cured, but apart from the blood of Jesus there is no forgiveness of sins.

You must do all within your power to prevent homosexuality in your children. But you should also teach your children that God loves and desires to redeem all sinners, including homosexuals. One of the most outstanding and obvious characteristics our Lord displayed while on earth was His compassion. I believe He wants us to teach our children to treat homosexuals in much the same way as we are told He treated the woman caught in adultery in John, chapter eight. He understood that love, not judgment, has the greater likelihood of producing true repentance in people.

Single Parents and Sexuality

Single parenting is no doubt one of the most difficult and demanding tasks that a person can ever confront. Earlier we discussed single parenting. A major concern for mothers raising sons alone is their boys' sexual development. The greatest fear many mothers have regarding their sons, concerns homosexuality. These mothers fear that in homes where the father is absent there will be an increased likelihood of homosexuality. In her excellent book *Single Mothers Raising Sons*, Bobbie Reed states that after much research she found no significant correlation between being raised by a single mom and being homosexual.[19]

We have already discussed the complicated and controversial theories related to the causes of homosexuality, and while mothers cannot be blamed for their son's sexual orientation, there are some things single mothers can do to encourage the development of a healthy sexual orientation. Here are a few suggestions:

1. *Provide good male role models for your son.* Moms need to work at finding good male role models for their sons. The key here is "good" role models. Coaches and other males can, unfortunately, often be negative role models. Strive to select positive male role models and use negative modeling situations as opportunities to teach. Do not attempt to be both parents.

2. *Avoid overprotecting your son.* Single mothers especially need to avoid overprotection because this practice tends to produce immature and overly dependent young men. This kind of dependence on the mother is believed to contribute to a homosexual orientation.

3. *Avoid excessively dominant behavior.* Mothers raising sons alone often feel the need to become very dominant. They

assume that boys need a firm hand and, since the father is gone, they need to become tougher and more dominant. Single mothers certainly need to discipline their male children assertively, but extreme dominance should be avoided. Several researchers believe there is a correlation between domineering mothers and homosexual sons. One study of homosexuals found that 76 percent had dominating mothers.[20]

4. *Encourage your son to develop a healthy attitude toward both sexes.* Single mothers should not criticize or belittle men in general. Your sons need to know that all men are not bad or evil. If boys are taught that men are evil creatures, how will they be able to accept their own manhood? Encourage your sons to have friends of both sexes, and to view both sexes as being capable of good and evil.

5. *Do not rely on your son to meet all your needs.* Single mothers sometimes consume all energy and time their sons have, in an effort to meet their personal needs. Mothers must branch out and become involved in a variety of activities, and free their sons to develop healthy attitudes and activities.

So far we have confined our discussion of single parenting to mothers raising sons. Single parents, again mostly mothers, must also rear daughters. Most mothers, however, feel more confident in this role because they know from experience how girls should act and feel. But single mothers of daughters should also avoid certain pitfalls. For example, a mother should not overly criticize men, especially her daughter's father. In order for young girls to develop healthy attitudes toward men they must not be exposed to constant criticism of males. The importance of a father figure for teenage girls has already been established. The single mother should encourage a good relationship between her daughter and the child's father. If such a relationship is not possible, then mothers must seek positive male substitutes (grandfather, uncles, youth ministers, etc.).

The subject of single parenting is much too complex to be totally discussed in this book. We are focusing on sex education and the promotion of healthy, godly sexual attitudes and orientations. In seeking to prevent premature sexual activity and to avoid a homosexual orientation, it is of paramount importance for single parents to live sexually and morally pure lives. A wholesome example of godly attitudes and behavior will have more influence on children than any other single factor. When parents are striving to live according to God's will and plan, children will not fail to notice or emulate this attitude.

Single parents, like all parents, need to provide wholesome, godly sex education for their children. The principles contained in this book can be taught and practiced by single parents. Your task will be more difficult because you will not have anyone with whom to share the work and the stress of sex education. But plunge ahead and when additional help is needed find sources for such help. For example, do not hesitate to call upon ministers, counselors, relatives or anyone who can teach and demonstrate healthy sexual attitudes to your children. Ask the Lord to provide help—He has promised to provide!

For Further Thought

1. What specific plans do you have to inform your children about STDs and AIDS?
2. In your opinion, should teenagers be provided with factual information regarding birth control? If you told your child that premarital sex is wrong, but if they choose to engage in such activity they should protect themselves—do you believe such a statement gives a "double message"?
3. How does your child feel about birth control and "double messages"? How can you find out?
4. What are your attitudes and feelings regarding abortion? Is abortion an option when rape or the life of the mother is in danger?
5. Write a letter to your teenager explaining your feelings about abortion. Deliver the letter and use it as a discussion starter.

6. What prejudices prevent you from viewing life as sacred and dignified?
7. Ask your children to recall the last time you asked for their forgiveness.
8. Ask your child to define homosexuality (if he/she is old enough). What are the sources of his/her information?
9. Ask your son if he has ever worried about being homosexual. Ask why.
10. Discuss "homophobia" with your teenage children.
11. Do you believe God will forgive homosexuals? What would need to be involved?
12. If you are the single mother of sons, make a list of possible male role models for your son.
13. Ask your child (adolescent or preadolescent) whether you are overprotective. If he says yes, ask for an explanation.
14. Relate some of your fears as a single parent to your children. Discuss them.
15. Read John 8:1-11 with your children. What relevance does this passage have to your thoughts about abortion, homosexuality, etc.?

Chapter 12

FINAL
THOUGHTS

Being able to provide accurate, honest sexual information in an atmosphere of openness and caring represents the ideal goal of sex education. However, in the real world the ideal often does not happen. Many parents have the desire to provide sex education for their children but lack the skills or resources necessary to do a thorough job. Other parents are simply not comfortable discussing sexual matters. I believe that parents can do an effective job of sex education when the desire and the resources are available, and hopefully, this book will have provided some of these resources. There are many other good books available to assist you. However, the greatest resource available to you should be the church.

The Church's Role
Our churches must begin to become actively involved in the sex education of our children. Many parents object to sex education taught by the public schools because such teaching

generally ignores the moral and spiritual aspects of sexuality. Therefore, logically, churches should help provide sex education resources to families. Providing sexual resources and help for parents during the coming decade will be one of the church's greatest challenges. It could also be one of the church's greatest legacies. Churches can assist families with regard to sexual matters in several ways. Here are a few possibilities:

1. *Provide sex education classes for families.* Ideally, trained ministers and counselors should teach parents how to provide sex education in the home and should help parents to create the open environment so vital to sex education. Churches should have regular, ongoing classes designed to equip parents with the necessary skills to teach effectively on all sexual matters. Churches should also have sex education courses specifically designed for children of all ages, especially adolescents. Sex education taught by trained church personnel would complement what is being taught in the home. Children would be receiving moral and spiritual teaching on human sexuality at church, and then having such teaching reinforced at home by additional teaching and demonstration. Such repetition of godly teaching is necessary to offset the constant bombardment of sexual material heaped on children by the media.

   Many issues would need to be negotiated and settled before a church could begin a program of sex education. These include: At what age do the classes begin? At what age do both sexes attend the same class? How do you handle the more controversial issues? and many others. But offering such classes to families should be a high priority for churches. Of course the involvement of the parents would be necessary from the beginning. It has been my experience that when parents are involved and communicated with, they will support such a program.

   A youth minister friend of mine organized sex education classes for junior high student in an effective and nonthreatening manner. On Sunday nights the class material would be presented to the parents. The parents had an opportunity to hear, experience and discuss all the issues that were to be presented to their children. Then on the following Wednesday evening the material would be taught to the junior highers. This schedule encouraged parental participation and involvement, while at the same time providing needed sex education to the students. Church leaders and parents cooperated for the benefit of their children. You must insist on this kind of help from your church. And if help is not forthcoming, you may have to find another church that will assist you in providing biblical sex education for your children.

2. *Provide a library of resources.* Churches should maintain a library of helpful books, periodicals, audio and video tapes, and other resource material. There are many helpful books available on the subject of sex education. Many parents will check out and use helpful resources when these are available. When sex education classes are being offered it helps to have the material available for parents to look at. After examining the curriculum, parents will feel more at ease and will probably be more supportive.

3. *Provide parental support groups.* Churches should encourage and organize parent support groups on a variety of issues. When functioning properly, the church is a supporting community of believers who sustain and serve one another. Support groups consist of small numbers of parents who are either presently experiencing, or have experienced, similar situations and circumstances. Such groups meet regularly to encourage, serve, support and love one another. Hurting parents benefit greatly by being part of a group that understands and listens.

The sexual sins of a child usually produce a tremendous amount of guilt in Christian parents. As a result of this guilt and accompanying embarrassment, parents will probably not voluntarily join a support group advertised as being for parents with sexually active children. Church leaders must be creative and subtle in providing help for hurting parents.

For example, our church has regular, general parental support group meetings called HELP (Help, Encouragement, and Learning for Parents). At these meetings discussion on a prearranged topic encourages participation by all parents of adolescents. These parent meetings have two purposes: to provide help, encouragement and peer support for parents in a nonthreatening and genial environment, and to encourage parents with specific adolescent problems to seek help from the appropriate group.

In other words, when parents begin attending the HELP meetings and the staff discovers, or the parents admit specific problems, they can be directed to functioning support groups designed to deal with the specific problem. When handled sensitively this procedure integrates hurting parents with others who have had similar experiences, and it also avoids public embarrassment. Most churches are full of parents who have experienced painful problems with their children. Some of the parents have successfully solved these problems and others have learned from their mistakes. Many are very willing to encourage and help others who are having similar struggles. Such sharing, encouraging, listening and supporting helps parents survive difficult struggles with their children. As Christians we are to "bear...one another's burdens" (Gal. 6:2, KJV).

If your church is not large enough or does not have trained staff to assist with support groups, perhaps you might cooperate with other churches in your area to offer this needed help. In addition, there are parachurch organizations in many cities that provide parental support groups. You can obtain information about parent support groups by calling youth ministers, counselors, pastors and other church leaders. Hopefully, your church already has a support group helping parents cope with sexual, as well as other adolescent problems, but if not, perhaps you can help start such a program. The benefits of parents helping parents are great, and parental support groups should be a high priority of churches.

4. *Provide professional counseling.* Many churches have trained counselors as part of their regular ministerial staff. These skilled professionals can provide much needed counseling during times of crisis. Hurting families receive many benefits when churches offer this service. Churches that lack the means to furnish staff counselors can help families with adolescent problems in at least two ways. First, the church staff could include a qualified youth minister. Most youth ministers have some training in counseling and can deal effectively with most typical adolescent problems. Often the most beneficial counseling resource youth ministers can provide involves helping parents determine when professional counseling assistance is needed. A qualified youth minister should be able to differentiate between normal transitional adolescent problems and deviant behavior that requires the services of a professional counselor.

Churches can also help families with adolescent problems by developing a working relationship with Christian counselors in their area. Pastors, youth ministers and other church leaders should be familiar with local counselors and psychologists. This contact will help church leaders direct families to the appropriate professionals. Good Christian counselors who combine professional training with adherence to God's principles are valuable assets to parents struggling with major adolescent problems.

5. *Provide an active, effective youth program.* Youth programs can help teenagers remain sexually pure by surrounding them with a positive peer support group, and by offering programs that minimize sexual opportunities and encourage group activities. I have already mentioned the positive effects of a supportive Christian peer group. Teens who are part of a loving, active and serving Christian youth group have an easier time resisting sexual temptation.

The youth ministry program can assist teens in avoiding

sexual misconduct in at least two ways. First, the program should emphasize sound biblical teaching regarding sexual issues. Biblical teaching on sexual matters should be integrated into the Sunday school curriculum on a regular basis and can also be very effective as a part of retreat or camp programs. This kind of teaching will help negate the onslaught of sexual stimulus teens receive from society.

A second way that the youth program can help teens avoid sexual problems relates to specific activities within the program. For example, youth activities that promote one-on-one boy/girl relationships, especially among young adolescents, should be discouraged. Instead, activities

> The church can, and must be, the special place
> where our children learn about sexuality, and
> where they receive protection and help as they
> learn to cope with their sexuality.

should be structured around groups of boys and girls. Activities must also attempt to avoid pushing young boys and girls together before they are old enough for such relationships.

I have mentioned the situation that arose at our summer camp, where somehow the tradition of taking "dates" to our final evening bonfire began with the older campers. Before long, through pressure and example, we had third- and fourth-grade girls devastated because they did not have a date to the bonfire, or because they had a date with the wrong person. No one on our staff encouraged or anticipated this problem. Youth ministers must not only plan activities that avoid boy/girl relationships for those too young, but they must also actively organize and promote activities that stress group dating.

Churches also need to find ways to provide their young people with positive peer pressure. Christian teens need to function as support groups, helping each other stand up against the enormous sexual pressures of today's society.

The church can, and must be, the special place where our children learn about sexuality, and where they receive protection and help as they learn to cope with their sexuality.

Fear Versus Lordship

Many of the good books available today on the subject of teenage sexuality or sex education contain large sections devoted to the reasons teenagers have sex, and reasons they should not have sex. These books, and the particular sections that concentrate on causes and prevention, are excellent resources. I have, however, deliberately chosen not to include such lists in this work. There is perhaps some benefit derived from examining causes, but in order to help teens effectively to avoid premarital sexual involvement, parents must begin early teaching and demonstrating wholesome, godly sexual values and attitudes. When Christian values, attitudes, and accurate information are provided in an atmosphere of openness and love, children will be much less lively to succumb to sexual temptations. Our energy should be concentrated on providing positive, ongoing sex education for our children.

This book was written as a resource designed to help you as you attempt to help your children avoid sexual sin. Hopefully the principles stressed here will help you teach your children about human sexuality from a Christian perspective. Unfortunately, too many parents fail to provide early sexual training to their children and later, when the children reach adolescence, the parents attempt to use scare tactics and fear to prevent sexual activity. The use of fear becomes a substitute for continual and accurate sex education.

I am not saying that teenagers should not be warned about the possible consequences of sexual sins. They need to know that if they engage in sexual intercourse devastating consequences are a possibility. They need to know that even though God forgives sin, He does not remove the consequences of sin. God will forgive sexual sins, but if pregnancy occurs, there will be a baby nine months later. But after seventeen years of working directly with teens, and helping rear two teens of my own, I am convinced there is only one sure antidote for sexual promiscuity: the Lordship of Jesus Christ.

It is appropriate to use a certain amount of healthy fear to help your teens avoid sexual involvement. Tell them that if they are sexually active, possible consequences might involve pregnancy, AIDS, sexually transmitted diseases and other physical and emotional problems. However, avoid the temptation to use fear as the only or primary teaching method. This distorts the biblical message of true sexuality. Begin early

---

Providing honest, accurate sexual information within the framework of an open, caring family is one of the most important parental responsibilities of our age.

---

in the life of your children to teach the concept of the Lordship of Jesus. Christian teens need to be taught to avoid sexual sins because they have given their lives to Jesus. The apostle Paul says in 1 Cor. 6:18-20:

> Flee from sexual immorality. All other sins a man commits are outside his body, but he who sins sexually sins against his own body. Do you not know that your body is a temple of the Holy Spirit, who is in you, whom you have received from God? You are not your own; you were bought at a price. Therefore honor God with your body.

Teenagers need to be taught to avoid sexual activity because they have been "bought at a price." Their bodies have been purchased and house the Holy Spirit of God. They flee sexual sins because of the tremendous hurt such activity causes their Lord. My experience as a parent and a youth minister tells me that adolescents can understand and relate to this message when it is lovingly and continually taught and demonstrated to them.

And, of course, providing children with accurate and honest sexual information is of critical importance in today's society. We live in a time of great sexual awareness, and a time of almost total absence of societal restraints and morals. Frances Schaeffer in his book *Whatever Happened to the Human Race?* says, "Aldous Huxley said it clearly in his brilliant little novel *Brave New World.* In it he pictures a society which has reversed the morality of the present, especially in the area of sexual relationships. Faithfulness within a unique love relationship becomes evil; promiscuity becomes good."[1] Providing honest, accurate sexual information within the framework of an open, caring family is one of the most important parental responsibilities of our age.

It is my prayer that God will help you teach your children about this beautiful gift of sex.

NOTES

Introduction
1. Josh McDowell and Dick Day, *Why Wait?* (San Bernardino: Here's Life Publishers, 1987), pp. 22-24.
2. John Nieder, *God, Sex and Your Children* (Nashville: Thomas Nelson Publishers, 1988), p. 19.
3. David Lewis, Carley Dodd, Darryl Tippens, *Shattering the Silence* (Nashville: Christian Communication, 1989), p. 112.
4. McDowell and Day, *Why Wait?*, p. 40.
5. Donald M. Joy, *Parents, Kids and Sexual Integrity* (Waco: Word Books, 1988), p. XIV.

Chapter 1
1. Grace H. Ketterman, *How to Teach Your Child About Sex* (Old Tappan: Fleming H. Revell, 1981), p. 13.
2. Institute for Family Research and Education, *Community Sex Education Programs for Parents* (Syracuse: Institute for Family Research and Education), p. 3.
3. McDowell and Day, *Why Wait?*, p. 385.
4. Ibid., p. 384.
5. Candyce Stapen, "Speaking Frankly Isn't Being Permissive," *USA Today*, 3 September 1986, Nat'l Ed., p. 6.
6. Merton P. Strommen and A. Irene Strommen, *Five Cries of Parents* (New York: Harper & Row, 1985), p. 72.
7. Greer L. Fox, "The Family's Role in Adolescent Sexual Behavior," *Teenage Pregnancy in a Family Context* Theodora Ooms, ed., (Philadelphia: Temple University Press, 1981).
8. Institute for Family Research and Education, *Community Sex Education*, p. 44.
9. David Elkind, *The Hurried Child* (Reading: Addison-Wesley, 1981), p. 77.
10. Institute for Family Research and Education, *Community Sex Education*, p. 14.

Chapter 2
1. Josh McDowell, *What I Wish My Parents Knew About My Sexuality* (San Bernardino: Here's Life Publishers, 1987), p. 55.

2. Hershal D. Thornburg, "The Amount of Sex Information Learning Obtained During Early Adolescence," *Journal of Early Adolescence* 1.2 (1981) pp. 171-174.
3. "The Teen Environment." Based on a Study of Youth Strategies for Junior Achievement, The Robert Johnston Company, Inc., 1980, p. 4.
4. Strommen and Strommen, *Five Cries of Parents*, p. 115.
5. Cited in McDowell and Day, *Why Wait?* p. 40.
6. Tony Campolo, *Growing Up In America: A Sociology of Youth Ministry* (Grand Rapids: Zondervan Publishing House, 1989), p. 74.
7. Stewart Powell, "What Entertainers Are Doing to Our Kids," *U. S. News and World Report*, 28 October 1985, pp. 46-49.
8. Strommen and Strommen, *Five Cries of Parents*, pp. 78-79.

Chapter 3
1. Sol Gordon and Judith Gordon, *Raising a Child Conservatively in a Sexually Permissive World* (New York: Simon & Schuster, 1983), p. 90.
2. Institute for Family Research and Education, *Community Sex Education*, p. vii.
3. Sol Gordon and Craig W. Snyder, *Personal Issues in Human Sexuality* (Boston: Allyn and Bacon, 1986), p. 165.
4. Institute for Family Research and Education, *Community Sex Education*, p. 58.
5. Adapted from *Community Sex Education* (Syracuse: Institute for Family Research and Education), p. 58-63.
6. McDowell, *What I Wish*, p. 143.
7. Norman Wright and Rex Johnson, *Communication, Key to Your Teens* (Irvine: Harvest House, 1978), p. 110.

Chapter 4
1. Earl D. Wilson, *You Try Being a Teenager* (Portland: Multnomah Press, 1982), p. 65.
2. Strommen and Strommen, *Five Cries of Parents*, p. 88.
3. Ibid., p. 90.
4. Bruce Narramore, *Adolescence Is Not an Illness* (Old Tappan, NJ: Fleming H. Revell, 1980), p. 68.
5. G. Keith Olson, *Counseling Teenagers* (Loveland, CO: Group Publishing Inc., 1989) p. 65.
6. David Lewis, "Counseling Adolescents in the Church," Abilene Christian University Graduate Course, Abilene, 29 June 1987.
7. Olson, *Counseling Teenagers*, p. 65.
8. Kevin Leman, *Smart Kids, Stupid Choices* (Ventura, CA: Regal Books, 1982), pp. 113-114.
9. Fritz Ridenour, *What Teenagers Wish Their Parents Knew About Kids* (Waco, TX: Word Books, 1982), p. 162.

Chapter 5
1. Howard R. Lewis and Martha E. Lewis, *Parent's Guide to Teenage Sex and Pregnancy* (New York: St. Martins, 1980), p. 30.
2. Letha Scanzoni, *Sex Is a Parent Affair* (Ventura: Regal Books, 1973) pp. 36-37.
3. John Nieder, *God, Sex and Your Children* (Nashville: Thomas Nelson Publishers, 1988), p. 83.

4. Lewis, *Parent's Guide*, pp. 36-37.
5. Ibid., p. 37.
6. James Dobson, "Focus on the Family", Family Convention, San Antonio, Sept. 1978.
7. Lewis, *Parent's Guide*, p. 44.
8. Ibid., p. 46.
9. Gordon, *Personal Issues*, p. 10.
10. Gordon, *Raising a Child Conservatively*, p. 45.

Chapter 6
1. Dorothy L. Williams, ed., *Yes You Can! A Guide for Sexuality Education that Affirms Abstinence Among Young Adolescents* (Minneapolis: Search Institute, 1987), p. 39.
2. Mary Ann Mayo, *Parents Guide to Sex Education* (Grand Rapids: Zondervan, 1986), p. 124.
3. Gordon, *Raising a Child Conservatively*, p. 27.
4. Ketterman, *How to Teach*, pp. 93-94.
5. Ibid., p. 94.
6. Scanzoni, *Sex Is a Parent Affair*, p. 130.

Chapter 7
1. Mayo, *Parent's Guide to Sex Education*, p. 142.
2. Williams, *Yes You Can*, p. 107.
3. Donald M. Joy, *Bonding* (Waco: Word Publishers, 1985), pp. 127-28.
4. Paul D. Meier, Frank B. Minirth, and Frank Wichern, *Introduction to Psychology and Counseling: Christian Perspectives and Applications* (Grand Rapids: Baker Book House, 1982), p. 116.
5. Bobbie Reed, *Single Mothers Raising Sons* (Nashville: Thomas Nelson Publishers, 1988), p. 135.
6. Jean Lush, *Mothers and Sons* (Old Tappan: Fleming H. Revell, 1988), pp. 75-79.
7. Williams, *Yes You Can*, p. 108.
8. Olson, *Counseling Teenagers*, p. 28.
9. Grace Ketterman, *Depression Hits Every Family* (Nashville: Thomas Nelson, 1988), pp. 168-170.
10. Gordon, *Personal Issues*, p. 117.
11. Gordon, *Raising a Child Conservatively*, p. 84.

Chapter 8
1. Gilman D. Grave, *The Control of the Onset of Puberty* (New York: John Wiley & Sons, 1974), p. xxiii.
2. McDowell, *Why Wait*, p. 56.
3. Ketterman, *How to Teach*, p. 122.
4. David Elkind, *All Grown Up and No Place to Go* (Reading: Addison-Wesley, 1984), p. 56.
5. Howard R. and Martha E. Lewis, *Sex Education Begins at Home* (Norwalk: Appleton-Century-Crofts, 1983), p. 43.
6. Wayne Rice, *Junior High Ministry* (Grand Rapids: Zondervan, 1987), p. 63.
7. Kevin Leman, *Smart Girls Don't and Guys Don't Either* (Ventura: Regal Books, 1982), p. 19.

8. Elkind, *All Grown Up.* p. 57.
9. Ronald L. Koteskey, *Understanding Adolescence* (Wheaton: Victor Books, 1987), pp. 80-81.
10. Mayo, *Parent's Guide to Sex Education* p. 180.
11. Charles Shedd, *The Stork Is Dead* (Waco: Word, 1968), p. 73.
12. Earl D. Wilson, *Sexual Sanity* (Downers Grove: InterVarsity Press, 1984), pp. 63-64.
13. James Dobson, *Preparing for Adolescence* (Ventura: Regal, 1978), pp. 86-87.
14. Kevin Leman, *Smart Kids, Stupid Choices*, p. 29.
15. James Dobson, *Dr. Dobson Answers Your Questions* (Wheaton: Tyndale House, 1982), p. 93.

Chapter 9
1. Thornburg, *Journal of Early Adolescence*, pp. 171-72.
2. Strommen and Strommen, *Five Cries of Parents*, p. 59.
3. Williams, *Yes You Can*, p. 14.
4. Leah Lefstein, "A Portrait of Young Adolescents in the 1980s," Center for Early Adolescence, University of North Carolina (1986) p. 7.
5. John McDowell, *How to Help Your Child Say No to Sexual Pressure* (Waco: Word, 1987), p. 22.
6. Elkind, *All Grown Up*, p. 166.
7. Leman, *Smart Kids*, p. 47.
8. Olson, *Counseling Teenagers* pp. 75-76.
9. Barry and Carol St. Clair, *Talking with Your Kids About Love, Sex and Dating* (San Bernardino: Here's Life Publishers, 1989). p. 100.
10. Koteskey, *Understanding Adolescence.*, p. 101.
11. Olson, *Counseling Teenagers*, p. 38.
12. Wilson, *You Try Being a Teenager*, pp. 120-21.

Chapter 10
1. Scott Kirby, *Dating* (Grand Rapids: Baker Book House, 1979), pp. 34-36.
2. Norman Wright and Marvin Inmon, *Dating, Waiting and Choosing a Mate* (Irvine: Harvest House, 1978), pp. 145-46.
3. Campolo, *Growing Up in America*, p. 84.
4. Ibid., p. 85.
5. Grace H. Ketterman, *199 Questions Parents Ask* (Old Tappan: Fleming H. Revell, 1986), p. 209.
6. Charlene Walker, Lecture on Teenage Pregnancy, Abilene Christian University Graduate School, Abilene, Texas, 1 July 1987.

Chapter 11
1. Gordon, *Raising a Child Conservatively*, p. 165.
2. Lewis J. Lord, "Sex with Care," *U.S. News & World Report*, 2 June 1986, p. 53.
3. Leman, *Smart Kids*, p. 64.
4. Gordon, *Personal Issues*, p. 185.
5. Gordon, *Raising a Child Conservatively*, pp. 174-75.
6. Ibid., pp. 174-75.
7. Deborah Schmook "Aids," *Waco Tribune-Herald*, 21 Feb. 1988, early ed., B1.
8. Margaret Rosenberg, *Issues in Focus* (Ventura: Regal Books, 1989), p. 40.

9. Gordon Golden, M.D. (Doctor of Internal Medicine and member of AIDS Task Force in Texas), Lecture on Aids, Abilene Christian University Graduate School, Abilene, 2 July 1987.
10. Ibid.
11. Gordon, *Raising a Child Conservatively*, p. 92.
12. Stephen R. Jorgensen, "Sex Education and the Reduction of Adolescent Pregna cies: Prospects for the 1980s," *Journal of Early Adolescence* 1.1 (1981), p. 43.
13. Lewis, *Parent's Guide*, p. 33.
14. Institute for Family Research and Education, *Community Sex Education*, p. 19.
15. Francis A. Schaeffer and C. Everett Koop, *Whatever Happened to the Human Race?* (Old Tappan: Fleming H. Revell, 1979), p. 113.
16. Olson, *Counseling Teens*, p. 423.
17. Wilson, *Sexual Sanity*, p. 91.
18. Nieder, *God, Sex and Your Child*, p. 181.
19. Reed, *Single Mothers Raising Sons*, p. 133.
20. Lush, *Mothers and Sons*, p. 106.

Chapter 12
1. Schaeffer, *Whatever Happened to the Human Race?* p. 136.

GLOSSARY

Abdomen - The lower part of the trunk of the body (belly).

Abortion - The expulsion of a human fetus (unborn baby). An abortion may result from natural body function (miscarriage) or it may be done intentionally by a doctor at the mother's request.

Adolescence - From the Latin "to grow up." The state or process of growing from childhood to adulthood. Generally the years between 12-19.

Adrenal - One of a pair of glands located above the kidneys. They produce hormones which help control body metabolism.

Amnion - The sac in which the baby is contained inside the uterus.

Anus - The opening at the lower end of the alimentary canal, through which solid waste passes.

Areola - A ring of dark color around the nipple of a breast.

Bisexual - One who is sexually responsive to or aroused by both sexes.

Bladder - A sac or organ in the pelvic cavity for the storage of urine.

Cesarean section - A method of delivery by surgical procedure in which a baby is taken through an incision through the walls of the abdomen and uterus. This procedure is done when the mother cannot have a normal vaginal delivery.

Cervix - The neck or constricted lower end of the uterus which leads to the vagina.

Chromosome - Small particles of protein substance that are found in a cell nucleus, and which carry the genes in a linear order.

Circumcision - The surgical procedure of removing the loose skin (foreskin) from the end of the penis.

Climax - The high point of excitement in sexual intercourse (orgasm).

Clitoris - A small, sensitive organ located just beneath the lower edge of the pubic bone where the inner folds of the vulva meet. With stimulation it becomes rigid and erect and causes muscular contraction extending to the vagina. When stimulated it is extremely pleasurable to the female. It is similar to a tiny penis.

Coitus - The act of sexual intercourse between two human beings.

Conception - The beginning of the organism that grows into a baby. This happens when a sperm attaches to the ovum and fertilization takes place.

Condom - A thin rubber sheath worn over the penis during sexual intercourse to prevent conception or venereal disease.

Contraception - The prevention of conception either by preventing the sperm and ovum from meeting, or by destroying their ability to fertilize. Birth control.

Copulation - Sexual union or intercourse.

Douche - The process of cleansing or washing the vagina with water or disinfectants.

Ejaculate (Ejaculation) - The discharge of semen from the penis.

Embryo - An organism in the earlier stages of its development. In humans it refers to the fertilized egg during the first eight weeks of growth in the uterus.

Epididymis - An elongated tube on the back of the testis (testicle) where the sperm are stored until they travel into the body.

Erection - The condition in which the penis stiffens and becomes rigid. This happens as blood fills tissue during sexual arousal. The penis in this condition is ready for sexual intercourse.

Estrogen - The primary female sex hormone that is partly responsible for breast development and other feminine traits.

Fallopian tubes - A pair of slender hallow tubes connecting the womb and the ovaries. The egg is released by the ovary and through gentle movement of the tube the egg travels to the uterus.

Fertilize or Fertilization - To make pregnant. The union of the male sperm and female ovum.

Fetus - In humans, the developing baby from the beginning of the third month until birth.

Foreplay - Sexual stimulation, usually including hugging, petting, kissing, caressing or rubbing, intended to create sexual arousal and lead to sexual intercourse.

Foreskin - Loose skin covering the head of the penis. It can be removed by circumcision.

Frigidity - The inability of a person to enjoy or respond to sexual stimulation. Usually applied to the female.

Gene - Complex part of a chromosome that determines a person's uniqueness. Genes are responsible for color of eyes and hair, facial features and other traits.

Genital - Pertaining to the sexual organs. Used as a plural noun, "genitals," it means the reproductive organs, especially the external sex organs.

Gland - A group of cells or an organ that produce a secretion. Some glands eliminate waste (sweat gland), others secrete substances which affect growth and development (pituitary, adrenal, thyroid, ovary and testis).

Glans penis - The head of the penis.

Gonads - The reproductive glands (ovaries and testicles).

Homosexual - A person who is sexually aroused by, or who satisfies his or her sexual desires with a person of the same sex.

Hormone - A chemical substance or compound produced by a gland and transported to a specific organ of the body to stimulate and regulate the activity of that organ. Different hormones affect different parts of the body.

Hymen - A fold of mucous membrane that partially closes the entrance to the vagina.

Impotence - The inability of a male to achieve an erection, which results in being incapable of functioning sexually.

Incest - Sexual intercourse between close relatives or family members.

Intercourse - Sexual coupling (coitus). Intimate physical closeness between a husband and wife. The husband inserts his erect penis into the wife's vagina and through thrusting movements a climax or orgasm is reached. The husband ejects semen and unless preventive measures are taken, pregnancy may result.

Labia (plural of labium) - Lip-like folds of skin bordering and protecting the vagina. The labia majora are sometimes called the outer lips, and the labia minora, the inner lips.

Labor - The contraction of the walls of the uterus as the baby is slowly pushed through the cervix and through the vagina. Labor may last from a few hours to an entire day.

Lesbian - A female homosexual.

Masochism - A perversion in which sexual gratification depends on suffering physical pain and humiliation.

Masturbation - Stimulation or manipulation of one's own genital organs, often to the point of orgasm. Sexual self-gratification.

Menarche - The beginning of a female's menstrual cycle. It generally occurs approximately one year after the appearance of body and pubic hair.

Menopause - The period of permanent stoppage of menstruation in women, usually occurring between the ages of 45 and 50. Ovulation stops and pregnancy is no longer possible.

Menses - The periodic flow of blood and tissue from the uterus.

Menstruation - The monthly discharge of blood and tissue from the uterus, occurring approximately monthly, from puberty to menopause. This tissue lines the womb in preparation for the growth of a baby, and when conception does not take place it is discharged.

Miscarriage - The expulsion or birth of a baby (fetus) before it is able to survive. Usually occurs between the third and seventh month.

Navel - A depression or low area in the middle of the abdomen at the point where the umbilical cord was attached to the placenta.

Nocturnal emission - (wet dream) - The passing or automatic discharge of semen and sperm from the male during sleep. It is experienced by most adolescent boys as a normal way nature releases sexual tension.

Orgasm - The climax or peak of sexual intercourse, accomplished by high excitement and followed by a sense of relaxation. In males the ejection of semen occurs with orgasm.

Ovaries - Two reproductive glands of a woman, located in the lower abdominal region. These glands produce tiny eggs (ova) and sex hormones.

Ovulation - The formation and discharge of mature eggs from the ovary to the fallopian tube. Generally occurs every 25-30 days.

Ovum - The female reproductive cell (egg) formed in the ovary. The singular of ova.

Penis - The male genital or sex organ through which urine and semen pass out of the body. An erect penis is normally about five to seven inches in length and one-and-a-half inches in diameter.

Pituitary - A small oval gland attached to the base of the brain. It secretes hormones regulating growth of the body and the activity of other glands.

Placenta - The organ formed in the lining of the uterus by the union of the uterine mucous membrane with the membranes of the fetus. It serves to feed the baby and to dispose of waste. The umbilical cord connects the placenta and the baby.

Pregnant - The condition of having a baby developing in the body. The process of nurture and growth of a fertilized ovum in the uterus generally takes nine months (280 days).

Prepuce - The fold of skin that covers the head of the penis (foreskin).

Prostitute - A person who engages in sexual intercourse for money.

Prostate gland - A gland at the base of the bladder, surrounding the urethra, which secretes a fluid that becomes part of the semen.

Puberty - The age at which a person begins rapid physical development and becomes capable of reproduction. It generally occurs between 13 and 16 in boys and between 11 and 14 in girls.

Pubic - Related to the lower part of the abdomen, where hair grows.

Rape - The act of physically forcing a person to have sexual intercourse against that person's will.

Rectum - The lower end or terminal section of the large intestine, extending to the anus.

Sadism - A perversion in which sexual gratification is gained through causing physical pain or humiliation.

Scrotum - The external sac of skin and muscle fibers in which the testicles hang between the male's legs.

Semen - The thick whitish fluid produced in the male reproductive organs, containing sperm and discharged through the penis. It is produced in the testicle for fertilizing the female ovum.

Seminal vesicle - Two small storage sacs near the urinary bladder and prostate. The sperm cells and seminal fluid are stored here after production.

Smegma - A thick secretion that collects beneath the foreskin or around the clitoris.

Sperm (spermatozon—plural is spermatozoa) - The male sex cell which fertilizes the female ovum (egg) and is produced in the testicles. It is about the size of a pin point and is shaped like a tadpole with a head and tail. It contains genes and chromosomes which are needed to create human life.

Sterile - Incapable of producing offspring.

Sterilization - A process whereby a man or woman is made sterile or unable to produce children.

Testes (plural of testis) - The male reproductive glands (gonad) suspended in a sac between the legs. These glands produce sperm.

Testosterone - The predominantly male sex hormone secreted by the testicles that stimulates masculine characteristics.

Testicle - One of the two male reproductive glands. They produce sperm.

Thyroid - A gland located in the front of the neck. Its secretion regulates the rates of metabolism and body growth.

Umbilical cord - The cord which connects the baby to the placenta within the uterus and through which the baby is fed.

Urethra - The membranous tube through which the urine passes from the bladder to the exterior. In males it also carries the discharge of semen.

Uterus - A muscular hollow organ of the female reproductive system in which the fertilized ovum implants itself and develops into a baby. During the growth of the baby it stretches and expands.

Vagina - The passage connecting the uterus with the outside of the body.

Vas deferens - The duct or tube that transports the sperm from the testicles to the penis.

Virgin - A person who has never had sexual intercourse.

Vulva - The folds of skin, flesh and other structures which protect the opening of the vagina.